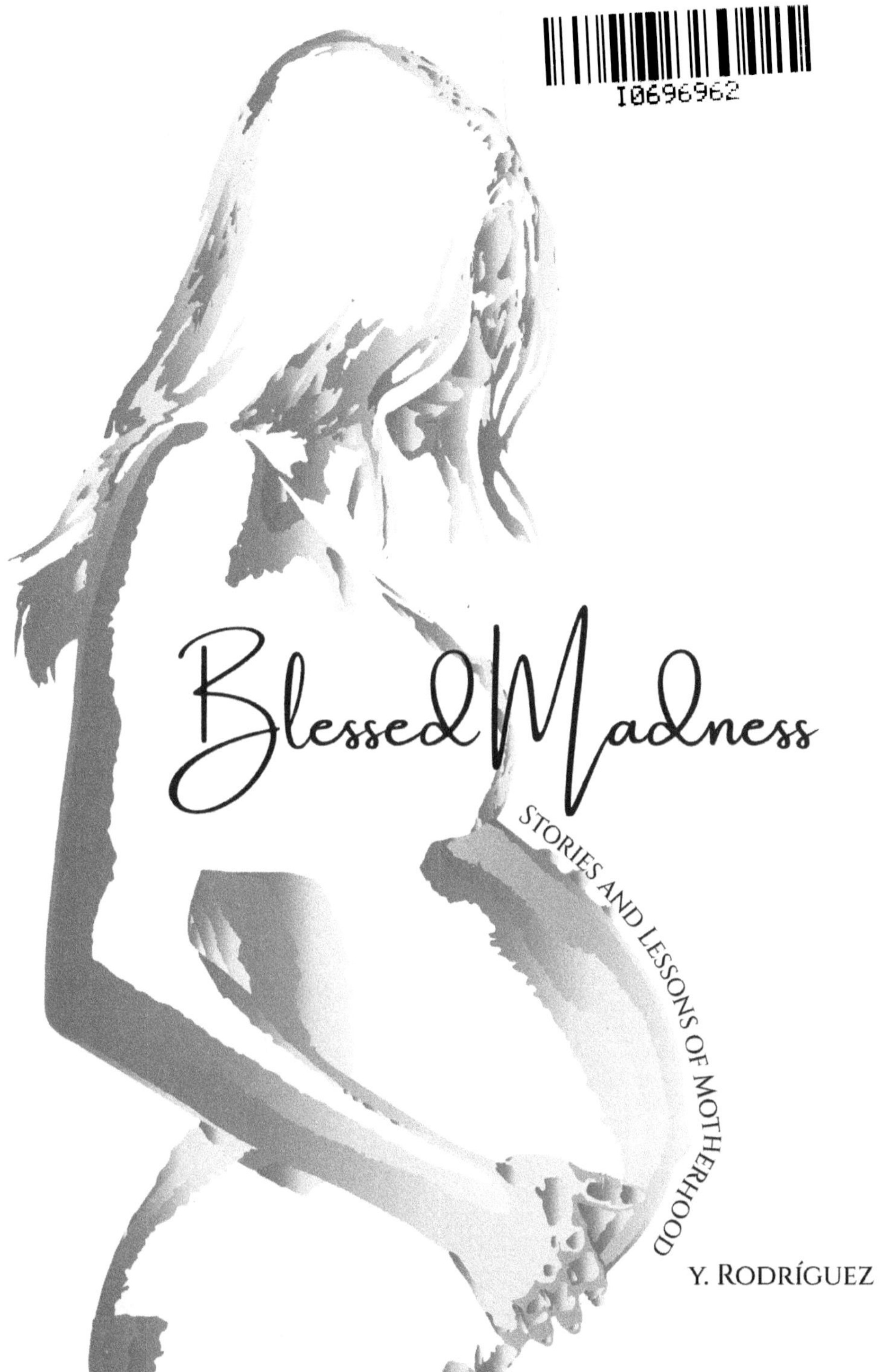

I0696962
Blessed Madness
STORIES AND LESSONS OF MOTHERHOOD
Y. RODRÍGUEZ

DEDICATORY

To Ariel, for the challenging adventure of motherhood.

Índice

ACKNOWLEDGEMENTS

To my sister, because she turned the impulses expressed in these chronicles into a real book that can help many families around the world.

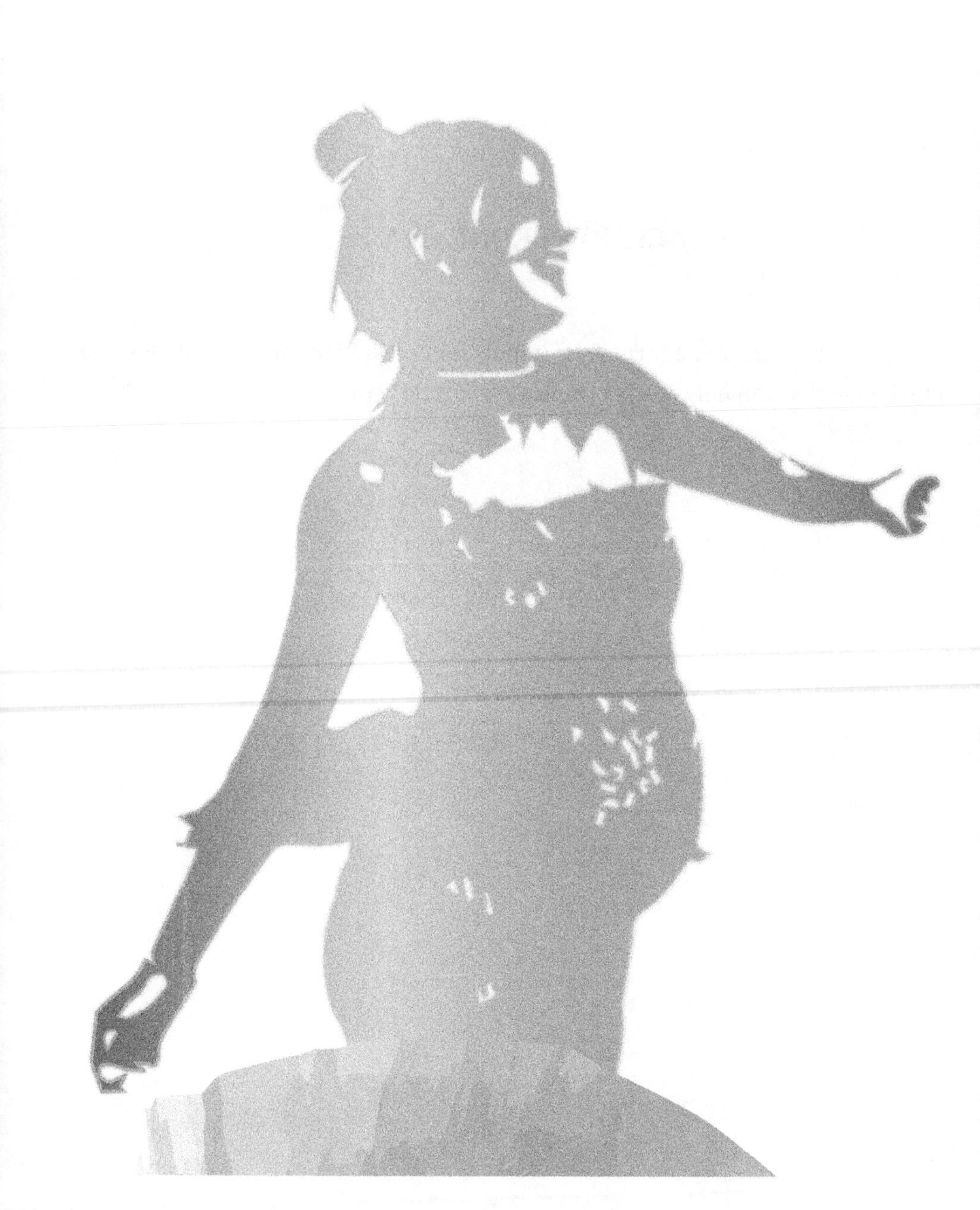

Chapter 1: About Doctors Appointments and Hospitals

When we decided to have a baby

This November marks one year to the day since my husband and I decided to expand our family. We had been married since June and had been together for two years.

I know people from other generations, might seem this like a rash decision, since our relationship was short compared to other eras. However, I don't think those who share our age will find it weird.

Nowadays, a love relationship is measured not so much by years, but by passion. And that is our case. Little time, a lot of passion and the conviction that we should prove to be more than two.

That's why, after almost nine years using a contraceptive that allowed me to finish college without "unwanted surprises", and great part of the exercise of my profession in different media press, I went to the family doctor's office and asked her to withdraw it.

Now, with my 29 years old, I knew there was such a thing as "family planning"… a medical service based on counseling couples who want to have children, so I asked the doctor to explain what we should do. She did. And we complied.

 However… December, January, February, March… and nothing happened.

I always thought that the day I decided to have my own babies, everything would be very easy. I come from a very fertile family, with plenty of uncles, cousins, second and third cousins on both my mother's and father's side. Since it is also a long-lived family, I have the opportunity every day to appreciate the family tree in its full extent and vitality.

That's why I was so worried when in March we had not yet achieved insemination.

It's been only three months, my friends said, but it is difficult not to worry when you are surrounded by questions such as: will we be fertile?, maybe we have no "chemistry"?, maybe something is wrong with us?, how long do we have to try?...

Then came the time for the suggestions. One of my friends sent me an application to my mobile phone that could calculate the fertile days of each month and the chances of fertilization resulting in a boy or a girl.

A few days later, I don't remember if it was Maria, my husband's neighbor (almost a grandmother), or someone else in the family, who suggested that we should experiment with some "traditional methods", like preparing güira honey[1]. This is a concoction that women in Cuba drink in the belief that it "prepares the womb". There was no harm in trying it. We bought the honey and were looking for the güira when... my menstruation stopped.

I am a punctual person, even with my periods, so the first day I was late, I took a pregnancy test. I had saved the test for a year. Fair and square, it was overdue, but I didn't care. Whether it worked or not, I would end up going to the doctor for an ultrasound and a baby.

The two positive lines came up immediately. I didn't even have to wait the regularly required minutes, as instructed by the doctor. And at that moment, the house was filled with fireworks.

Medical records and other stories

I am 36 weeks pregnant. A week more or less doesn't make any difference. Next Thursday, when I turn 37 weeks, my baby will be ready to come into the world.

In the meantime, I'll tell you how we've been doing...

To get to the end of a pregnancy, a pregnant woman in Cuba has to go to countless medical appointments. Mine were all in Marianao, one of the most populated municipalities in Havana. The area where my Family Doctor Office is located is

---

1   Güira honey: concoction of the Cuban Traditional Medicine, prepared with the pulp of the güira (natural tree of Tropical America, fruit of the same name), honey and rum. It has a high content of vitamin E and although it does not have proven therapeutic effects, it is popularly used in the treatment of bronchial asthma and respiratory conditions, as well as to increase fertility in women and the success in the conception. (Note from the editor)

popularly called "La Finca" (The Farm) because from there almost everything is woods, and bush and green …. and the streets are not streets, but roads. It is also an unhealthy area where hundreds of people live, most of them, as the doctor would say, with a low level of education.

My doctor, strangely enough, is not Cuban. I had never been treated by a foreign specialist, which is what my doctor is, although he has been living on the island for 10 years and knows all the intricacies from top to bottom of our oral and body language. Hector came to Cuba to study medicine and is about to finish his Specialty as a General Practitioner, so then he can start Cardiology, his true passion.

He probably won't even know my baby after dealing with him these 9 months of pregnancy, because in December he'll be finishing with us to start dealing with patients suffering health problems more related to the heart.

Above the Doctor Office lives Valentina, the doctor's right hand.

Speaking of hearts, Valentina is the heart of the office, the neighborhood, the district, and probably the whole area surrounding "La Finca". She has worked there as a nurse for 30 years and has seen many specialists pass through the small medical office. She knows all the children in the area, having taken care of their mothers during their pregnancies, and she has helped every elderly person. With her special way of being, she knows how to convince those who run away from a vaccination or a cytological test.

Valentina has never left. And when she disappears for any reason, personal or professional, patients/friends miss her immediately.

A few months ago, she was transferred to a nursing home for a few days. An experienced nurse was needed. But the family practice almost collapsed. There are many things besides injections that a nurse can do to ease the burden off the doctor's shoulders.

I didn't know that until I saw the office full of people who just wanted their blood pressure checked, to know if their labs had arrived, a prescription for recurring ailments that didn't warrant "stealing" minutes from the doctor, an update on a medication card, a cytology test, to ask a question, the phone number of pharmacies in the area, help with a bedridden person, advice on a medication, a diet that was probably already signed and stamped, or of course their daily injection...

Can you imagine the picture? It was chaos.

On the contrary, my first visit to Hector that November was unusual. There was almost no one there. The doctor came by the house to tell me that it was time to see him and that I should leave in two hours. "without fear, because it seemed that people were already feeling the festive spirit of the end of the year," he told me.

I don't know if in other countries a doctor would take the trouble to visit every pregnant women's house or other fragile patients in his area, but here they do.

The thing is, when I arrived at the office and saw that there were only two people waiting, I decided not to take advantage of my "pregnant privileges" and waited patiently for my turn.

In 20 minutes, Hector's voice asking for "the next one" told me to go in for what would be the longest medical consultation of my entire pregnancy. ....

The longest medical consultation

Hector, my family doctor, is good, but "a little slow," they say. According to the neighbors who frequent the office, this speed is because "he is not Cuban", although - in their opinion too- the Bolivian is not lacking in sparks.

The truth is that Hector is not slow, he is meticulous. Every person he treats is a serious matter for him, whether it is a cough or a case of cancer. Being so, every patient takes a long time…. especially pregnant women. This philosophy is something they teach in the Cuban Academy.

Since I know him, and I think 9 months is enough to learn a doctor's style, I try to be the first person in line whenever it's time for my regular visit with him. I never succeed. I always have Margot in front of me.

Margot is an old lady who must be between 80 and 90 years old. I always find her at 7:00 a.m. sitting on the steps leading up to the nurses' home above the doctor office, waiting for Valentina to open the doors so she can move from the stairs to one of the "orthopedic" chairs inside.

A considerable hump crushes Margot, who suffers from severe back, waist, and hip pain, which is why she wears a very tight girdle and why she visits Hector so often. I ran into her so many times that I have memorized his biography.

She is from the Sierra Maestra[2], where she helped the rebel army during the war against Fulgencio Batista, who was president of the Cuban Government until January 1, 1959. She had two of her children in the countryside where she lived, and two more in Havana, where she came to live and work with her husband. Not all of her children live in Cuba. And although she lives close to her daughters, who take care of her every day, she lives alone. She is an independent woman who works at the same Retirement Home where she says she goes because she is entertained and protected.

---

2   The Sierra Maestra is a mountain range in the southeastern region of Cuba mainly in the provinces of Granma and Santiago de Cuba (Note from the editor)

When we meet, Hector, out of consideration for my pregnancy, insists that he must see me first... but then I look at Margot, so old, with this huge hump, with this long history, with this loneliness that is and is not loneliness, and I feel sorry for her. And I let her go first with the doctor. Anyway, I'm not going to give birth right there... and I feel fine.

In the last consultation I had, I was neither the first nor the second person in line. I was the third, too far back for my taste and patience, even though the wait was only 20 minutes.

Hector came by my house around 8:00 a.m. to let me know that I should come see him for a pregnancy checkup since I was in the last few weeks of my pregnancy. He also warned me to come in two hours "without fear, because it seemed that people were already feeling the festive spirit of the end of the year," he said.

When I arrived, not surprisingly, I didn't see Margot. Not that I thought about her, because her visits to the doctor office start very early, but Valentina told me that the old lady had had an accident at home. She had a broken hip.

Poor Margot, I thought, even though my mother insists that you shouldn't call anyone "poor" or "poor thing". But I couldn't help it: in addition to the hump and the pain, Margot would probably need a wheelchair now...

Then I heard Hector's voice say "next", so I went in for my pregnancy checkup. And that, despite the emptiness of the office, was my longest medical interview.

He opened my medical record, which is almost a book and decorated with a small Chinese doll that Valentina got from who knows where, and began to write on a blank piece of paper: November 6, 2018.

He hadn't finished the second line, which began with "Pregnant women with 35.5 weeks..." when an elderly, dark-skinned man with a bunch of onions in his hand entered the office on the verge of fainting.

The office consists of four small rooms: the doctor's office, a room for naked examinations and vaccinations, the bathroom, a small area that smells like a laboratory, where medicines, sterilized cotton and syringes are kept, and finally the waiting room, where you get to know Cuba through personal stories, mixed with this or that illness.

"Doctor", whispered the gentleman from the waiting room, so that Hector would come out to see him. And he did, but not before apologizing to me. The man had felt weak, out of breath, and like he was about to fall to the floor. The doctor took his blood pressure twice, just in case, and said, "He's fine". He auscultated his chest and back and again said, "He's fine". He asked him to open his eyes and looked at his pupil with the cell phone flashlight, but found nothing. In a lower tone, sitting next to him, he said something I couldn't understand, and Valentina accompanied him to his new destination.

"I know what he has", he said enigmatically as he returned to his table and didn't speak any more about the matter, which seemed serious despite the several "ok's" I had heard.

He immediately instructed me to get on the scale, the most terrifying of pregnancy moments. Then "get on the table to measure your belly, let's see how the baby is doing, let's listen to the baby's heart, I'll help you up, let's go back to the table…"

– Is the child moving? –he asked, feeling my legs and feet for swelling.

– Yes, very much, it keeps me awake– I replied.

And the doctor quickly wrote down the data of the physical examination. In the middle of the page, another pregnant woman entered the office and Valentina's voice, asking what was wrong, interrupted my consultation.

The new pregnant woman, 22 years old, felt contractions. She went straight to the doctor. She didn't even sit down.

Hector, amazed at the visit of the girl who should have gone directly to the Maternal Hospital as she was instructed, observed, as in the previous 37 weeks, her extreme thinness, and asked her if she had been to the hospital. "Yes", she said, "but since I still have contractions at intervals, I was allowed to come home. I live nearby, and the beds for admissions are full until 8:00 p.m.", she replied. The doctor insisted that she should have stayed at the Maternal Hospital, to which she stubbornly replied no, and that all she needed now was an indication for the calculation of the baby's weight, which they had asked her for at the Hospital. Hector gave it to her. She left.

Two interruptions. The medical consultation lasted more than an hour, and we were not even halfway through.

I tell the doctor to hurry up. He laughs, it is not the first time he has been told that. He still have to "comment" on what the gynecologist's weight calculation showed 15 days ago, and that he must translate it for me, because there's no one who can understands the doctors' handwriting, not even the ones of those who do ultrasounds.

And he starts to write, until a new commotion comes from outside his small office.

This time it was a woman in her forties, unhappy with the results of the hemoglobin analysis that Valentina had just given her, informing her that everything was fine. The lady, who obviously is very familiar with the doctor, interrupts and says that she only wants to see one small thing.

"Please, Hector, you must indicate me another blood test, this result doesn't convince me. It says 12 and they say that the hemoglobin does not show such a rapid increase," she pleads, standing up. Hector replies that "this is exactly why these tests are usually done three months after the start of treatment, although it could be that this result is fine."

"What are you taking or eating?" he asks, and I, who listens to everything, already understand that this is another consultation within the consultation, so I'll be out of there around noon, hopefully...

The woman rambles on about her diet until finally, at the doctor's insistence about the composition of her medications, she admits to be taking "buffalo liver" supplements. The doctor smiles. "Your test results are fine", he says. "Offal is the food that raises hemoglobin the most."

The self-medicating woman apologizes and leaves, but not before complimenting the doctor.

I look at him again, with a "hurry up" accompanied by "next time I'll assert my pregnant privileges," which elicits Hector's third apology in two hours.

"See you on the 20th", he finally says, and I, between tired and grateful, only manage to say "To send me to the Maternal Hospital, right?

Scheduled cesarean section

A C-section is a serious matter. And yet… all the girls seem to want it. It's like the Holy Grail of Motherhood in Cuba.

Some spend the 9 months of pregnancy trying to secure this operation. They make friends with specialists in gynecology and obstetrics in the maternity hospitals, they call family members and friends who are graduates in any medical specialty to accompany them at the time of delivery, and they can go so far as to pressure the doctors who assist them with spoiling behavior, insults, or threats.

At 36 weeks of pregnancy, I have only met two pregnant women who refused a C-section.

The first one was during a genetics consultation, and to the arguments of those around her commenting on the pros and cons of the natural birth, a girl responded firmly that the female body is prepared for vaginal delivery…not so for surgery. The other one had had two previous experiences that were "very fast", "with pain, but not too bad" and in her opinion "the better the mother behaves, the better she is treated".

But in most of the stories that one hears in the waiting rooms of doctors' offices, polyclinics and hospitals, the anecdotes that abound are different….

Pregnant women whose babies had "fetal distress" because the doctors waited until the last second of the last possible week to subject them to a cesarean section, pregnant women with dilations of 10 centimeters from which the baby still could not come out, babies who changed position during contractions, induced dilations that lasted more than 24 hours with the pain that this entailed, and many other experiences closer to terror than to what you could expect of something "normal", "natural", "very own of the female body", and that women have been doing since "the beginning of time". …

There is a whole popular theory about how a woman about to give birth in a Cuban hospital should and should not behave in order to be treated condescendingly by the doctors.

If you cry and scream a lot, they will ignore you. If you insult and threaten, they will ignore you. If you are weak and feeble, they will treat you harshly. If you make them angry, they make you wait longer than you should. Behave well, they tell you, to sum up.

And with all this going on in your head, you wonder if it wouldn't been better if they take you straight to the operating room. Then, perhaps, the well-being of the baby and its mother would not depend so much on the temperament of the patient and the doctors … according to the vox populi. Although, according to the doctors, the more upset a woman is at this crucial moment in her life, the less cooperative she is and the more she delays every step of the process.

In the case of cesarean sections, not all the stories are complacent. "I was left with remains inside", "I could not have any more children" and "the wound is terrible"… are some of the associated criteria.

When I was 34 weeks pregnant, my gynecologist, Margarita, predicted a dystocia delivery because of my severe scoliosis and the pain in my back. Of course I googled it. The word "dystocia" is not something you hear every day and it means something like problematic, with probable medical intervention, perhaps a "planned C-section". The gynecologist referred me to an orthopedist.

Margarita is an experienced and kind doctor. She rotates by my doctor office every 15 days and takes each pregnant woman with problems to her heart. On my first consultation with her, when I was 14 weeks pregnant, she had to see a 14-year-old teenager who was more than 7 months pregnant before she could see me. The girl was accompanied by her father, who said that the girl's mother happened to notice the protrusion of the child's belly. The girl gave birth naturally.

I always thought I would have a C-section. I spent 7 years of my life with a cast corset on my spine and hips. Orthopedic specialists had warned me about the likelihood of problems during childbirth.

Now Margarita says that even though the orthopedist suggested a C-section and she has scheduled it, there is a one percent chance that it will not happen.

The obstetricians of the maternity hospital have the last word.

Genetic

Few things can make your brain go blank. One of them, during pregnancy, is genetic consultation. There is such a good chance that the baby has a hereditary health problem that any suspicion stops your heart.

The first time we had such a consultation was at 12 weeks of pregnancy. Héctor, the family doctor, told us that we would have to attend a series of six specialized consultations, considered "essential" in Cuba, as part of the Maternal and Infant Program, which monitors the health of every pregnant woman and her baby.

So, for the first time in my life, accompanied by my husband, I met with an obstetrician-gynecologist, a clinician, a nutritionist, a psychologist, a cardiologist (whom I saw again at 26 weeks of pregnancy) and a geneticist.

I am not exaggerating when I say that the visit to the last one was the most exhaustive. So much so that, although I did not see her again during the entire pregnancy, I will follow the indications she wrote in the medical record on May 7, 2018, until my baby is 5 years old. The conversation with her was almost like a police interrogation. She wanted to know everything. And I told her everything.

Fortunately, we came out unscathed.

No risk had seemed too great to her. Not the family history of diabetes and hypertension, not my father's death from a stroke, not the first cousins on both sides of the family with Down syndrome or deafness. Nothing.

- "Although", she said, "the final word will come with the genetic ultrasounds".

The remaining three consultations were at the Genetics Center in Marianao. It was there that we saw our baby for the first time, through the monitor, and not without some anxiety, because the specialists, aware to the ignorance of the future parents, explained what they were looking for in each scan.

I still remember the second ultrasound.

I was 22 weeks pregnant and Dr. Gisela was puzzled by the baby's position. The baby didn't let her see what she wanted to see, so suddenly she said, "Get up and walk around, let's see if that activates and moves him a little". I went back. Nothing. "Go and eat something". I went back. Nothing. "Ask the nurse for a cold pack".... And that, apparently, was too much for the baby. When I came back, he had turned so much that in less than three minutes the doctor saw the lips and the heart, what she was finally looking for.

After the third ultrasound, at 30 weeks, I was discharged. The report said: "No major anomalies were observed, although those that do not show up on ultrasound or appear later cannot be ruled out".

We left relieved...even though we didn't like that last warning.

When you think about genetics, you tend to focus on what the child will look like, or what traits you may or may not want it to inherit. But during pregnancy, you learn that's not the most important thing. Doctors teach you that health comes before aesthetics, and that's why they focus so carefully on every organ and length of the baby.

However, I have one recommendation for them:

Please think of another way to place the ultrasound monitor. We, expectant mothers, are the only people in those little medical rooms who don't get to see the little one... It inspires and cheers us up, especially when there is no paper to print the classic little photo.

Prepare for the hospital

I don't need a C-section, at least for now.

This is what the deputy medical director of the Maternal Hospital in Marianao told me. I had been told to see her after going to the Term Pregnancy Consultation, where I had been referred by the gynecologist, because the orthopedic who attended me during my pregnancy had recommended a C-section with a medical certificate.

Since my spine was in a cast from the age of 11 to 18, still have more than 40 degrees of dorso-lumbar deviation, and I had severe back pain during my pregnancy, it is normal that the orthopedist took his precautions.

However, according to the deputy medical director of the hospital, this pathology is subject to cesarean section only if the patient presents a treatment with steel rods or other complications, from which, fortunately, I am exempt. "All this means", she clarified, "that I will have a natural birth unless some exceptional circumstance leads to a different decision".

That being the case, I am now ready to feel the contractions...

Staying in a maternity hospital in Cuba is not something that the girls I have met tell me is pleasant. When they talk about it, they don't go into detail. For them, and I think it will be the same for me, the moment of arrival and departure was more important.

But for the closest grandmothers that my baby will have, the arrival and departure are as important as the preparation, taking into account the characteristics of the hospital in Cuba. For this reason, and because I had nothing better to do, I spent almost two weeks packing my bags to go to the medical center.

What should I take with me to the hospital? How do I know how many days to prepare for? According to doctors and anecdotal evidence, the average hospital stay for a newborn baby and his mom is about three days for a natural birth and up to seven days for a C-section.

Not all cases are the same, and there is always the possibility that some complication may prolong the obligatory stay.

However, there are some elements that should not be missing in the luggage of a pregnant woman and her baby.

This is what mine contains:

Mom's luggage

- Five lightweight, affordable outfits for breastfeeding my baby.

- Outfit for leaving the hospital

- Underwear

- Sanitary pads

- Flip flops

- Daily toiletries (soap, toothpaste, toothbrush, shampoo, skin cream, comb, deodorant, etc.)

- Frequently used medicines (prenatal, folic acid, dipyrone, vitamins, etc...)

- Bathing bucket and table fan (these items must be brought to Cuban hospitals)

- Sheets and pillow

- Cutlery and glass

Baby's luggage

Three Cradle Diapers

Oilcloth sheet for the crib mattress

Crib mosquito net

1 package of 1st stage diapers

Bundle of warm clothes to leave the delivery room plus the diapers

A change of clothes for leaving the hospital

10 bodysuits to spend the days and nights

A big bottle with boiled water to bathe the baby

Toiletries for the baby.

It is always possible that some products, both mine and the child's, will run out before we get home. To avoid collective schizophrenia in such moments, it is good to have a Plan B, which consists of having a duplicate at home of the products that can be used up.

That way, in the event of any shortage, you will only inform the family that accompanies you on what you need and where it is.

Seven things nobody tells you about pregnancy

And here I am, so annoying, to tell you what all pregnant women probably forget once they stop being pregnant. Because holding a baby in your arms has its magic, and so does pregnancy... although not all the time.

I didn't suffered from vomits, so I'll leave that bad experience out of my list and just stick to what I felt. Hope you find it helpful.

A small pregnant belly can be a problem.

If you are between two and five months pregnant, you may feel insecure about your rights as a pregnant woman in Cuba. You may not know whether to ask for the yellow seat on the bus, or that when the bus is full, no one will offer you their seat because they think you are a big person. In the queues, you're hardly a priority because your belly doesn't look big yet. I always carried my pregnancy card in my wallet... just in case.

A big pregnant belly can also be a problem.

Although a big belly usually generates good feelings in others, the truth is that it also causes setbacks. Adapt: Not everyone will look at you with a good face, especially the city bus drivers who will have to wait patiently for you (and they lack patience) while you get on and find a seat. Nor will those standing in lines where you are given priority, not even physically disabled people, because they will see it as a bad thing that others are trying to give you priority... because of course you are not sick. Be strong and demand your rights without being ashamed.

Eating and weight will be torture.

It doesn't matter if you are at the right weight or, like me, overweight: what you eat and how much you eat will be a frequent topic in almost all of your medical consultations. The weight you gain becomes a ghost that haunts you every hour. If you don't eat well, it's a problem because you shouldn't lose weight.

If you eat well, it is a dilemma because you should not gain too many pounds. And be careful, during pregnancy it sometimes seems that you are gaining weight even though you are not eating that much.

The medical consultations will interfere with your professional life.

You may think that it is possible to have a pregnancy while working. I share this idea, but you will find that it is not an absolute truth. Even if you feel fine 90% of the time during the 8 months you will be working before you go on maternity leave, there will be times when you will need to take a break from work:

medical exams for all three trimesters and extra exams if your doctor thinks you need them;

biweekly consultations with the family practice doctor

Consultations with specialists in genetics, gynecology, nutrition, clinical, psychology, and cardiology. If, like me, you have back pain, add orthopedics to the list;

Maternity licence.

Your baby's movements may not be so pleasant.

You imagine that, when you just start feeling the baby in your belly, he will be doing some somersaults. Or waving at you. But after 8 months, when he or she has more strength, the kicks in the ribs or belly can keep you awake...and even hurt a little. In my case, the baby does not stop moving when I am sitting or lying down. I can only get him to calm down when I'm standing...and it's impossible to stand all the time, so I'm getting used to him wanting to get out of my belly or not letting me sleep. I hope he won't be so naughty when he goes out...

Going to the bathroom will be your most recurring physical activity.

It's amazing how many times a pregnant woman can go to the bathroom during the day. For me, between 6:00 a.m. and 10:00 p.m., I go between 15 and 20 times. And I'm not lying! Be patient with yourself.

Being on maternity licence can be boring.

For those who are not used to being at home for so many hours, maternity leave can be a challenge. I left work at 34 weeks, as required by law.   I'm at 37 weeks and have nothing to do at home...except wait for the baby to be born.

All the household chores seem to be few and quick. And I don't have anything to prepare for my little one's arrival because I did everything the first week off so there, I didn't get bored at all! Advice? Make a list of the things you haven't had time to do and get to work. Remember not to do any intense physical exertion.

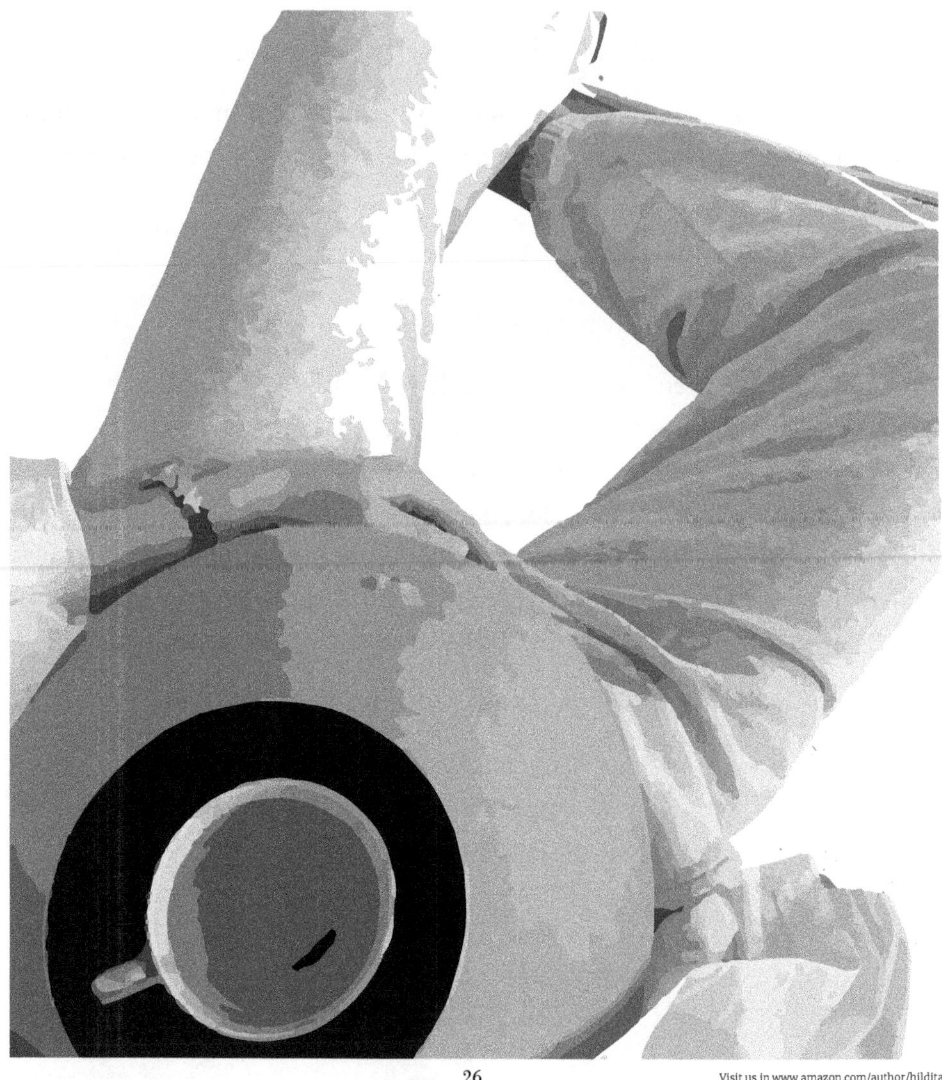

Chapter 2: Home Economics and Social Myths

Babies and low wages

How to prepare for the arrival of a baby when both parents work for a government institution in Cuba?

If you are a mother or a father and you belong to the sector I'm describing, you have surely asked yourself this question from the moment you knew the results of the pregnancy test or you knew about the first ultrasound.

The same thing happened to me. For the first two months, I racked my brain trying to figure out how to raise money, how to save money... while the on the way baby's grandparents melted with the desire to start buying the things Ariel would need.

The impossibility of doing so, due to the difficult correlation between the high cost of living and salary, prevented my husband and me from making much progress in this almost impossible mission.

And then the advices started pouring in:

- "A child comes into the world with a loaf of bread under his arm," was the comforting phrase of an elderly lady with cancer while waiting for one of the frequent doctor's appointments. Too bad it's not quite like that.

For the record, it is not that I go from doctor's office to doctor's office asking how those who are about to give birth to another human being make their living, but you hear a lot of things in the medical queues during the 9 months of pregnancy, and money is a recurring theme.

At other times, younger girls shared their experiences: some were supported financially by their parents; others by their families outside of Cuba or by their husbands, many of whom worked in the private sector; and a few I met - almost all of them over 35 - were financially independent enough to support their future babies, who were also their first children.

As you might guess, the latter pregnant women were my favorite stories.

They were women who had decided to expand their families when they already had professional and economic stability that made it easier... None of them complained that they were "too old," "too tired," or afraid of the "needle-in-the-womb test" that they must undergo after the age of 35 to ensure the health of their baby.

I am 30 years old. In these 7 years of work, I have never thought twice about trying new experiences in print, digital, radio or television journalism... inside or outside of Cuba. I love what I do... except that, unlike the 30-something women I've met, my salary is not enough.

In my experience, without a supportive and thoughtful network of family (or friends), it would be very difficult for a couple earning just over 500 pesos a month to meet the expenses of one child. Imagine two. Of course, this support network must be aware that help - financial or otherwise - does not mean that the parents are subordinating their primary role in the child's upbringing.

Based on my recent experience, I recommend that expectant parents not sit back and wait for help to "fall from the sky". There are actions that we can undertake ourselves, including not settling for just one job and opening a savings account.

Our generation is not like our parents' and grandparents', when a person focused on one job. That used to be enough to somehow support your family. But over the years, things have changed in Cuba.

Now young people are looking for flexible jobs, with schedules that leave time to earn a living in other ways (not necessarily in our professional profiles), and that facilitate the entry of the money needed to support the families we plan to create or have already created.

This option is offered by the state institutions, where it is possible to work as a contract worker, for a few hours a day... and also on the private sector.

The expansion of private work in Cuba has brought with it a wide range of new and old work options in which it is not necessary to be the 8 hours a day dedicated to the main state job that we do not want to quit. Some of these jobs can even be done from home.

I know that working two or three jobs is not a very accommodating alternative, but when you decide to bring a baby into the world, life changes, and as it changes, so do your comforts and priorities.

The power of a pregnant woman

A giant pregnant belly inspires feelings of solidarity… in theory. But I wouldn't put my hands in the fire to prove that hypothesis.

While I was not a pregnant woman, I always thought big bellies deserved every sign of gentleness. If you see them walking down the aisle of a bus looking for a yellow seat, you give them yours…even if you see that there is no sick or elderly person sitting in the yellow seat, even if you are a woman just like them, even if you are already an elderly person and deserve the seat as well. If you are standing and you see her, you do what every dignified person does: you raise your voice for her, so that those who occupy the yellow seats stand up.

Logic tells us that when pregnant, women are more vulnerable and everything is more difficult: walking, holding on, standing upright to keep balance, standing for hours, sitting for hours, spending time without eating, standing in line… in short, everything that anyone would normally do, even if they were a little tired or a little sick.

Not to mention that there are pregnant women who are hypertensive, diabetic, who suffer from severe headaches or spinal pain; pregnant women who do not stop vomiting during the 9 months, or who suffer from swollen limbs.

It is a pity that common sense has deteriorated so much.

When I was 16 weeks pregnant, I was scheduled for an ultrasound. In the queue, two visibly upset women objected to pregnant women being given priority just because of their condition when there were sick people there.

At the polyclinic where I was being treated, it was established that to be admitted for consultation, the order of the queue would be two people in line and a pregnant woman. The reaction of the women surprised me as much as the silence of some of the people present, especially those who would benefit from the unrestrained reaction, since they would logically see their appointments moved up. Fortunately, the doctor prevented it from taking on other dimensions.

At 25 weeks of pregnancy, I left work to take a bus that, as usual in Cuba, was packed with people. Since it was impossible to cross the aisle to get to the yellow seats because of the crowd, I decided to stay next to the driver, it was only two stops anyway. What did he say when he saw me? "You're in the way". I replied with an offer: "I'll get off and not go home... or I'll stay here". Embarrassed, he left me alone.

Another time, at 32 weeks, I went to the butcher to buy chicken. I would have liked my husband or mother-in-law to do this family chore, but it was my turn. In Cuba's butcher shops, pregnant women have priority. I don't know if it's a written law, but they have. So I go to the one in my neighborhood, I approach the line of the "plan jaba"[3] and I ask them please, if they can let me buy. None of the people responded, except an old woman who was the third and said: "If you want, behind me". I could have gone right to the front of the line and bought the chicken, but politeness always betrays me, so I replied, "So be it". And I bought after her.

The worst episode was when I was 34 weeks pregnant, with a very large belly.

On that occasion, I went to buy a bus ticket to go to Guantanamo with my mother. The lady at the door wouldn't allow me to buy both tickets, even though I explained that I couldn't travel alone because of my condition. She replied that after a problem with a pregnant woman who wanted to buy 7 tickets and caused an enormous reaction in the queue, the management of the Arenal Bus Agency had decided that the pregnant woman could only buy for herself and, if she had a child, for him.

I denounced their extremism and inflexibility. I asked to speak to the director of the agency or his second in command, but none of them had arrived and it was 10:00 a.m. Not knowing what to do, I told her that I would still wait in line, even if I only bought a ticket, which it would be of no use to me, but at least I could wait in case the bosses arrived. She told me to do it, but that nowhere was it written that bus companies should give priority to pregnant women, that it was a delicacy on her part. I have yet to find out his explanation...

---

3 Plan jaba: a system set up by the government to give priority to households where everyone works, when buying regulated products in the network of grocery stores and other food products (Note from the Editor).

Fortunately, that day, to my visible desperation and helplessness, an older gentleman, I think his name was Andres, told me to take the seat in front of him and buy as part of the normal queue. Immediately, a lady sitting in the corner of the hall jumped out and claimed that this was not fair, since I could buy the ticket for the destination she was traveling to and had been waiting for since 3:00 in the morning.

Andres, who had been there since 2:00 a.m., responded angrily but respectfully: "I will buy tickets for two other people and you, you should be ashamed of yourself".

Cheers, Andres. If it were not for you...

Parents

You can choose the father of your baby. However, you don't usually think about how good of a father your partner will be... Attraction overrides reason, and then security, love, and the certainty that living together can be a good idea take over. Then usually comes fertilization... although there are couples where the baby comes before any possible planning. I know several.

I chose my baby daddy.

Like many 30-something girls before me, I had other options, each of which faded with time. I was sure I hadn't found my stop until I met him. And then there are times in life when you have to say, "This is it".

The baby hasn't even been born yet, with my 37 week, and he's already a great dad. Of course, I didn't even know that was possible until I had my 8 pieces of irrefutable evidence:

Immense joy on the day he knew of the positive pregnancy test.

Her responsible accompaniment to each of the important medical appointments.

The enthusiastic and tireless way in which she took care of every little detail (light and huge) of preparing for the arrival.

His constant concern about how much and how I was eating.

The absolute understanding that pregnancy is not a disease, but a state of the body, and therefore the mother-to-be, also a professional, has the right to fulfill herself while the baby is forming.

His conscious assimilation of the meaning of the new reality when we were informed that we were having a boy and not a girl, as the whole family thought, except for my sister, who dreamed of having a nephew and taught him to play ball.

Preparing the wallet for future mishaps.

And his funny offers to "carry" the baby every time he sees me walking slowly and painfully because of this huge belly of mine.

When we began attending the almost mandatory medical consultations in Cuba at the beginning of pregnancy, the doctors looked with amazement at the presence of my husband next to me, listening to every detail as if he were "the pregnant one".

Each specialist had only one recommendation or question for him.

The gynecologist said that he only had to use protection during sexual relations, and the genetics specialist asked about the history of malformations in his family... although she specified that she was more interested in the mother-to-be, the clinician was only interested in his blood type... although it was mine that could give the bad note, the psychologist made known that his presence there was already a good sign, and the nutritionist called him to strengthen his pocket.

Summary? My husband concluded that fathers don't seem to be that important to doctors. Luckily for women, they are...although that has its pros and cons.

In these 9 months, I have had the opportunity to hear many stories. Most of them, from the mouths of other pregnant women, are about the dreaded moment of delivery...but others are about couples.

Future fathers who never were ok on the sex of the baby on the way, who left the relationship before the birth, who never took care of the baby, who heard "pregnancy" and ran away "from the picture"; men who were disengaged, transient...

Listening to these stories, one might think that perhaps the reason doctors focus so much on mothers is precisely because of these many anecdotes about fathers.

But then, in these days of waiting, you sit in the doorway of your house at 7:30 a.m. and see so many little children in uniform walking by, hand in hand with their fathers, carrying little backpacks of all colors, and you restructure your thinking: "there must be some scientific reasons, right? ....."

A Frankenstein for the pregnant woman

"In my time, in the middle of the Special Period[4], it was worse and I still had two children. Everything will be fine... just concentrate on the purchase of the essentials", recommended the mother of a pregnant woman in the health center of my community, in the middle of those debates with which we usually "kill" the waiting time in the queues... when people are in a good mood.

But what is essential when it comes to a baby? Or rather, what is not essential?

At the beginning of my pregnancy, a colleague of mine gave me a list of everything that "usually" completes a layette. Her list was a kind of "adaptable" inheritance, depending on the economic possibilities and the context of the pregnant woman who received it. My colleague had received it from a friend, who had received it from another, and so on. It is likely that the person who prepared it took elements from various Internet sites and created this kind of useful "Frankenstein for pregnant women".

When I received it, considering my family's particular financial situation, I couldn't help but be frightened. What a long list! I couldn't believe that a baby would need so many things. So my first thought was to prioritize:

Cross out everything that was not really "essential" according to my logic as a future mother/worker in the state sector.

Re-ordered what was left in order of priority. I basically put what I would need for the birth and the first few months. I left the list of medicines "in case..." last,

---

4   Cuba's peacetime Special Period was a long period of economic crisis that began as a result of the collapse of the Soviet Union in 1991 as well as the tightening of the US embargo since 1992. This period transformed Cuban society and its economy (Note from the Editor).

since almost all of them could only be bought in foreign currency in international pharmacies or brought from abroad... besides, "in Cuba it is always possible to take the baby to the pediatrician" -I thought- "whose consultation is free and who will recommend me cheaper medicines".

Give pieces of the list to interested relatives. Fortunately, there was the father, the grandparents, the aunt... all eager to collaborate.

Of course, as you might suspect, there was a mix-up somewhere along the way: socializing priorities.

Disposable diapers or cloth diapers? Bucket (for boiling diapers), pitcher (for boiling bottles), and aluminum pot (for preparing milk)? A crib bumper or just the three classic pillows to protect the baby? This many socks and tiny clothes? A diaper bag? A crib with or without drawers? A mosquito net for the stroller, the crib and the rocking crib? A baby carrier or just your arms? An inherited baby bathtub or a new one? Large or small towels? Crib diapers with or without embroidery? Everything new or not?!...

The debate is consubstantial to the Cuban family, so suddenly, what was for my mother and my mother-in-law a priority... including what wasn't used in their time; for my sister and me it was not essential. In the midst of my recurring inexperience and stubbornness, I saw it all very simply and - honestly - I think the baby would have survived the conditions I would impose on him.

Luckily... there was no need to do the test. To save the situation: everyone bought what they wanted.

When the time came - around 6 or 7 months - to buy the small layette that the state sells at a subsidized price to all pregnant women in the country, I had already almost completed mine.

Pregnancy layette

A soap opera with a lot of drama and action.

There is a popular myth in Cuba that you should not buy anything from the layette until you are six months pregnant. But almost no one follows it... the temptation is too great.

And one day, with 2 or 3 months of pregnancy, you find yourself accumulating first-stage disposable diapers and wipes... just in case they run out in the stores. A friend gives you bottles, clothes, a baby bathtub and a thermometer; an aunt buys you an irresistible toy; grandmothers show up with baby care products.... and so on until you get to the crib, sheets and everything else.

So... you go to the state store to see what the layette finally brings, which is sold to you at subsidized prices like the rest of the pregnant women of the nation, with the peace of mind that whatever it is, you already have almost everything. This is something extra, not fundamental, and fortunately!, because access to this layette can become a novel dilemma.

In the Marianao municipality of Havana, for example, the stores where they are sold are almost always out of stock, due to recurring problems in the production of the items that make up the layette.

Knowing the economic underdevelopment of my country and the constant economic crises that suffocate us, on the day of the purchase I went to the store aware that I would not find a crib, but what about the rest? The rest, yes, but not exempt from the unheard of.

First, since there was never anything in the store, the clerks decided to give all pregnant women the store's phone number to avoid the tedious and fruitless trips to the store. When it was time for my maternity leave, at 34 weeks pregnant, I started calling every day or two.

I had no time for it before, and now I had no luck finding a complete layette at the state store. Finally, one day, while waiting in line for an ultrasound to calculate the weight of the fetus, a discussion about the layette broke out, and a mulatto woman, obviously angry, said that she had gone to the Ministry of Commerce to analyze the situation in Marianao.

She was assured that the next day it would be sold the municipality's layettes corresponding that month.

- Are you sure?-I asked her.

- They have to be sure if they don't want a scandal- the girl replied, encouraged. She was 37 weeks pregnant and would be admitted for a C-section the following Monday.

I didn't call the store that afternoon. I just showed up at 8:30 a.m. To my surprise, I found a sign that said, "Closed for fumigation until 3:00 p.m." I never knew at what time they had fumigated the store, which opened at 9:00 a.m., or why they had to keep it closed so long instead of complying with the 45 minutes required by law, and finally fulfilling their social purpose. In the afternoon, I was informed that they would be selling the next day.

At 8:00 a.m. the next day, the line in front of the store was huge. As if in an absurd scene, at least thirty pregnant women, all more than six months pregnant and with very visible bellies, stood in front of the store in the sun. I was number 10, more or less. That's why I arrived so early.

Too bad that while I was waiting, I found out that not only would I be leaving without a crib, I would also be leaving without a crib mattress. ..... They hadn't arrived that month.

- So what are they selling? - I asked one of the first girls to come out of the store.

- Everything but the crib and mattress, a little crazy, you'll see, she replied.

And indeed. When you go in to buy, they ask you the sex of the baby.....

- Girl or boy? -they ask.

- Boy- I answer, because the colors of the package and the type of clothes will depend on it.

And the woman hands me a bag with sheets, boy's clothes and two pink towels! I pointed out that, as I understood it, the products for boys were blue or green. Yes, she argued apologetically, but the packers made a mistake and we can't change it. I looked at the shelf: there were hundreds of packages for girls with blue contents and just as many for boys with pink contents. Complete madness? Modernity?

Then they handed me a smaller bag, also pink, with perfume.

-Wrong again? – I ask.

-No –she replies– we only have these for now …. but you can wait for the boys'–.

I'm saving my energy for the crib mattress. Luckily I can wait up to a year for that, I said, thanking her and leaving.

Six hazings I paid for while pregnant

When you become a mother for the first time, it's hard not to pay for a little bit of hazing. This is my first pregnancy, so I guess you could say there were a lot of them. I will tell you about them... although I warn you that some of them are probably due to the particular circumstances of the health centers where I receive my care.

1. No privileges at my first appointment

The first time I went to the doctor for my pregnancy was for my "uptake"[5]. I had to go to work early, so, as I've usually seen, I asked for the last one in the line for the pregnant women. The nurse, who had never seen me before in her life since we had just moved into the neighborhood, asked me how far along I was. Twelve weeks, I replied. You're coming in for an uptake, she said, it takes a while, and since it's your first time, you'll have to stand in the regular line. I sat down and resigned myself.

2. Your husband does not benefit

There are many tests that a couple has to go through during the 9 months of pregnancy, but none is as exhaustive as the first ones. I remember that Hector, the family doctor, gave me 20 indications for tests and 5 for my husband. We went to the municipal clinic to have my blood drawn and, to my surprise, when I handed in my papers and his, the receptionist told us that my privilege in the queue was only for me, as a pregnant woman. He should ask for the last one in the normal line, even though we had arrived together and the tests were for the same reason. I was shocked.

---

5   In Cuba, pregnant women are included in the Maternal and Child Care Program from the first weeks of pregnancy to guarantee the well-being of pregnant women, postpartum women and children. (Note from the Editor).

3. You can be the subject of a practical medical lesson

There is a collective consensus that pregnant women look better in a dress, but practice says otherwise... until the moment when your belly is so big that you actually want to wear only the simplest clothes (the usual dress) and the least complicated shoes (the beloved flip-flops).

The thing is, in the doctor's office, while they are checking the length of your belly and other details, you may have a group of students watching your changing body. Doctors always try to cover the pelvic area while checking the belly, but to avoid unnecessary embarrassment, and if you already know that there won't be a vaginal exam, you can always attend consultations and ultrasounds wearing a pair of pants or leggings and a sweater.

That way, you can easily expose your belly, as much as the doctors may need. I learned this too late. By then I had anything to wear on the lower part my body.

4. If you don't take your leave in time, your income may be affected.

Since I felt absolutely fine when I reached 34 weeks of pregnancy, I discussed with my family whether or not I should take maternity leave at that time. It seemed to me that I could be more useful at the newspaper office than at home. Fortunately, they stopped me in time. It turns out that, according to the Labor Code, a woman has he right to be remunerated with a special calculation, the weeks ranging from the 34th week until the time of delivery. If you leave later than expected, you risk having your income affected.

My advice? Take the leave when it's due and, if you wish, continue to contribute to your work from time to time...on your terms, but don't lose what by right you're entitled to.

5. Don't eat sweets at night

I have always had a passion for sweets, but if there is one thing I would not repeat in a second pregnancy, it would be eating them at night. Every time I forget and eat even a small piece, the baby moves inside me so intensely and for so long that I can't sleep until the wee hours of the morning. I, being you, followed my advice.

6. Pelvic bones really hurt during the last few weeks.

Have you felt the pain that comes from squatting a lot? Well, that's how I feel now at 38 weeks. I didn't know the bones in my pelvis could hurt like this, which doesn't mean it's excruciating, but I can't deny that I spent weeks thinking I was sitting or lying the wrong way, until Mr. Google explained to me that the little pain means my body is preparing for natural labor. There's no solution to this, but I'm sharing it so you'll know.

Baby and Internet.

What a lucky boy Ariel is going to be! This December, the month of his birth, the Cuban Telecommunications Company fulfilled an old debt. Finally, all citizens of the country who want to access the Internet through their cell phones will be able to do so.

This means that, apart from the cost, his mother will not have to rely on others to publish the chronicles of his birth on this blog and that he will grow up widely connected. I hope that one day the problems of technological availability in my neighborhood will be solved so that we can have our landline phone back and access to Nauta Hogar[6].

For those of us who are or will be parents in Cuba, the expansion of Internet access brings challenges that the rest of the world has lived with for a long time: how to regulate children's dependence on technology and their inability to study or read beyond the first 10 results displayed by Google. They also need to be taught how to discriminate between news sources, how to counter information, and how to protect their privacy.

These problems did not exist when I was growing up. Back then, you had to go to the library and ask for a bunch of books until you found what you needed, and current events information was only available through national media channels. Citizen opinion was reduced to sending paper letters that only the addressee could read. In other words, the limits of knowledge and expression were greater.

I try to imagine myself going to the library to look up what a "grade III placenta" is, or "dystocia", or "contraindications in pregnancy"; and I do not imagine myself, because I know, safely and reliably, that all this is just a click away on the Internet.

---

6   In Cuba, Wi-Fi connection from home. (Note from the Editor).

When I was studying at high school, between 2003 and 2006, the only digital resource we had was the Encarta encyclopedia. Encarta was a multimedia application developed by Microsoft in 1997, and Cuba had massively used it in schools. It has not been updated since 2009, but it became one of the best-selling educational products in the world.

I found it boring and inadequate. Its articles on specific topics, with illustrations, audio, video and some games, could be gone through in a few days. Within a week you had nothing new to look for, unless you were a kid discovering the world.

I learned what the Internet was like 24 hours a day in college, between 2006 and 2011. During my freshman year, the network administrators would set up an email and internet account that rarely made it to the end of the month in megabytes. Almost like today's salary... And you could go to the computer labs day or night.

There was no wifi like today, but you surfed to exhaustion (yours and the megabytes), and from the many pages you read you took information home for schoolwork, although teachers were always worried about "copy and paste", especially from Wikipedia, a collaborative encyclopedia updated by millions of volunteers around the world, but unreliable.

In those days, if a guy with hacking skills (almost always from majors such as cybernetics or telecommunications) wanted to flatter a girl half addicted to the Internet, he would give her a list of stolen accounts and passwords. These courtships were dangerous...and you had to learn techniques to protect your passwords, especially when visiting computer labs of the computing major's students.

It never occurred to me during those years that I would one day connect from home using my cell phone. I didn't even have a cell phone until 2012... Although to buy a cellphone line become legal in 2008, Etecsa, the Cuban Telecommunications Company, sold them too expensive for my mother's income. Besides, what's the point in having one? - I told a friend one day - when I could always communicate with my family through landlines or public phones?

Now I can't live without my cell phone... and I despair at the inaccessibility of the Internet.

My child will not have this problem. It is even strange how this opening will not be too late for him, but at the right time. Family and friends will see him grow from other latitudes, he will be able to make friends all over the world, and he will have access to all kinds of opportunities for self-improvement.

He will also learn a lot, which is one of the great advantages of the Internet. Any doubt will be solved instantly. And he will be able to make his voice heard, publicly, from the most unusual platforms, if he have something to say to the world, because another of the great advantages of the Internet Network is that you end up being your own mean of communication.

Training for mommy and daddy

I saw in a movie that the best way to train for mom or dad is to take care of a tree or a doll that is treated like a baby. The goal was to keep them vital, and the protagonist of the movie had to follow pre-determined schedules of meals, sleep, and baths. The idea seemed great… until Thiago was born.

Having lived at home with only my parents, my sister and me all our lives - and my sister is almost as old as I am - the experience of living with a baby from its first days of life was foreign to me.

I think that's normal. When you are five years old and the one who follows you everywhere is four, you don't worry about helping someone to dress her or feed her… You are hardly satisfied with the fact that their toys and clothes are not the same.

With Thiago it was different.

My brother-in-law's little son was born when I was no longer living in my own house, but in my husband's… where we ended up, as in many Cuban homes, the couples of the male children of those who would become grandparents in 2016.

There were already six of us when the little boy was born, which ruined any chance that the cinematic proposal of the tree or the doll would work. Thiago absorbed everyone's attention, even mine, so devoted to working away from home.

Nights

My husband and I soon understood what it was like not to be able to sleep because of the baby's constant fussing and crying, because even when his mother was the one to respond, sometimes a late-night family gathering around the couch where we were trying to make him sleep, was inevitable.

Feeding

We learned that there are babies who love milk and others, like Thiago, who love yogurt; that Telesur[7] and the Mesa Redonda[8] can be entertaining audiovisual proposals for a child of months who is looking for entertainment; that a playpen is a good option... even if he still cannot sit or stand up, because it strengthens his muscles; and that rubber toys suitable for teething, as well as plastic bottles, should not be boiled for a long time... or they will melt. These last losses, a painful result of carelessness, we do not wish on anyone.

Toys

Forget the idea of having too many toys for the baby from birth. Thiago had too many, so many that he always ended up preferring the most abused ones, like an epic chicken that deflated and wouldn't let go, or some unusual ones, like cold water storage bottles, his shoes or the TV remote.

He didn't pay much attention to very sophisticated toys until he was about a year old. I remember a spinning top with lights and music that frightened him, even though it was designed to attract the attention of children his age. That doesn't mean he didn't like bright things, because cell phones and computers always piqued his dangerous curiosity.

The Language

When Thiago was two months old, I also took some lessons in infant language.

---

7   Telesur is a Latin American multi-state open television news channel, with headquarters in the city of Caracas, Venezuela (Note from the Editor).

8   A radio-television program performed as a round table, produced by Cuban Television. Debates are held between various experts to present, analyze and develop political, economic, social or cultural issues of national or international relevance (Note from the Editor).

I was obsessed with him learning my name before anyone else, so I started teaching him. And I succeeded... not without suffering. I learned, in this pitched battle that involved hours and hours of "conversation" with someone tiny with huge eyes who ignores you every two seconds, that despite many attempts, babies will say "mama" and/or "dada" first.

Thiago also said "Yisy" in his own way, but I suffered to achieve it. Fortunately, I was not the only one.

We tried unsuccessfully to teach him that Grandma Meylin was "Mima". He preferred to call her "mommy"...even though his little head got blocked when he tried to diminish the adjective to his mother. This last lesson was so confusing that at a certain point he called everyone he didn't know how to call "mommy," including his paternal grandfather and some uncles and aunts.

Grandma Marlen managed to get him to call her only "abue," while Wilfre - his grandfather - became "abuelo" after a few months. While he called Yohana, his maternal grandmother, by her first name, and no God could change his behavior.

Diseases

We also learned a lot about early morning fevers, vaporizations to get rid of bad colds, accidental bumps and bruises, and children's hospitals... reluctantly. It wasn't that Thiago was sickly, but every now and then something disturbed the peace of the household, and the slightest suspicion became a very serious matter to be discussed with the pediatrician.

Systems of Support

We uncles had the honorable role of "systems of support", something we never disliked, except when Thiago was sick, because it implied that he would be at the hospital, far away from home and from us.

The rest of the time we enjoyed it. Sometimes, even unnecessarily, his mother "paid" us with cookies and other sweets for the affection we gave the little one. But for the record, we would have taken care of him for free.

The afternoons and some nights with him allowed us to develop our techniques of feeding him and putting him to sleep, even against his will. We took the opportunity to encourage him to learn to walk or to make some mischief, we dressed him up, and sometimes we designed little games for him in which he always lost. His parents scolded us from time to time, but they understood how impossible it was to resist the charm of watching him strive to achieve each proposed goal.

Kindergarten

When he turned one, his parents took him to Maria to be cared for. Maria is the closest thing my husband and his brother have to a grandmother right now. She has over 40 years of experience taking care of children in her home. She runs her own kindergarten. And there's where Thiago started dealing with other nine children, both younger and older than him.

When I was allowed to take him there, I walked him the four blocks to the kindergarten. Walking a one-year-old that many yards can be exhausting. Thiago would stop every three steps, grab all the plants, look at everyone as if he had never explored that path before, and stray from the route at the slightest inattention. He would also get tired quickly and look at me with a "please carry me" face.

Every time Maria saw me holding hands with him, after smilingly calling me a "bully," she would reward him for the effort with a tight kiss. Maria was also one of the first names Thiago said.

A year later, he began attending the government's kindergarten for children, to which he quickly adapted, as if he had been born just to go to school and learn.

The farewell

Now Thiago is two years old, but he doesn't live with us anymore. We no longer have to bathe him, feed him, change his clothes, talk and play with him for hours on end, calm him down when he gets angry, or entertain him while his parents live other parts of their lives...

We see him when he comes to visit his grandparents, for a few hours or a night, and then all the experiences we have had with him become almost nothing when we see new skills in him.

He has learned to say his name clearly, knows all the family members by name, asks for what he wants, apologizes when he does something wrong, says thank you, knows all the objects in the house and identifies who owns what, plays with other children without shyness, falls and does not cry, eats by himself, has perfected his toilet training, and gives answers that one would not even suspect in his little head.

The only thing he hasn't learned yet is how to say what he did that day. ..... And thank goodness, because if he told his parents all the mischief things we did with him, we could be in trouble.

I saw in a movie that, fortunately, after the age of two, children lose the memory of the first months of their lives... When Thiago learns to tell what he remembers, I'll let you know if it's true.

Ariel, his name is Ariel

This is an article about identity.

Naming a person has transcendental importance... although many of us parents don't realize it until someone asks us why we named our children so. And there is always an answer.

The most common in Cuba is "I like it," but I like other explanations better.

My mom and dad's names don't have any great stories behind them. My mother is one of 17 children. With such a list of choices, Elsa was a good choice. My dad had 9 siblings, three of them boys, but his Elvis Ariel was not inherited by anyone in particular, at least as far as I know.

To change this tradition of rootless names, my mother gave me a little story along with my name.

The "Yisell" was chosen by one of my older cousins when she was 10 years old. Confusion followed the choice, and on the day of the birth registration, instead of being written "Giselle" as it should have been, the name was the victim of a creolization of which, who knows why, I am even proud.

My little sister's deserve more attention. Her name is Rosa Hilda. Rosa, inherited from one of my mother's many close sisters, and Hilda from my paternal grandmother, a sweet lady who died when we were not more than a decade old.

Now it was my husband and I's turn to choose a name for our baby.

At the beginning of the search, we knew what we didn't want: a novel name, just because.

If it was a girl– we told the family– we thought of Alexa. None of our relatives had that name, but it seemed appropriate[9]. We like the sound of it: impressive, accurate, and it honors his father's and my passion for technology. He is a computer engineer specializing in web programming, I am a journalist.

Of course, there was no shortage of jokes among our friends. Knowing us, some argued that we could have named him Google, or Samsung or Blue, alluding to the brands of some of the mobile phones used in Cuba. We all laughed.

When I was 26 weeks pregnant, I knew that contrary to all family predictions, based on how little my face and the shape of my belly had deformed, we would not have a girl... but a boy.

"Science" had spoken. And so the name search began again.

This time we couldn't think of any technological roots, so we thought of a figure we both admired for his good works. Fidel, my husband said, and I added Alejandro, which was his nickname in hiding.

Fidel Alejandro is good, inspiring... but, I told him days later, I would prefer his name to be Ariel.

Ariel was my father's middle name. It is a common name in my family. He had it, as did the youngest son of one of his brothers. When my father died of a stroke in 2004, one of my cousins also named her youngest offspring Ariel.

I only had my father by my side until I was 16 years old, but that time was enough to understand that he was an important person, not only for the small family that my mother, he, my sister and I formed... but also for his parents and siblings. He was from Maisí, a corner of Cuba that is still difficult to reach because of its

---

9   Alexa is a global tool, available on the Internet, works as a virtual assistant developed by Amazon, and with which you can interact through smart speakers (Note from the Editor).

complicated mountainous terrain, and where he always returned in search of his roots and to take care of those he loved. In the city we called him Elvis, in the country he was known as Ariel.

My husband agreed. He will be Ariel Alejandro, he concluded.

I just hope they don't make jokes about his name being the same as the Little Mermaid. Ariel is a unisex name.

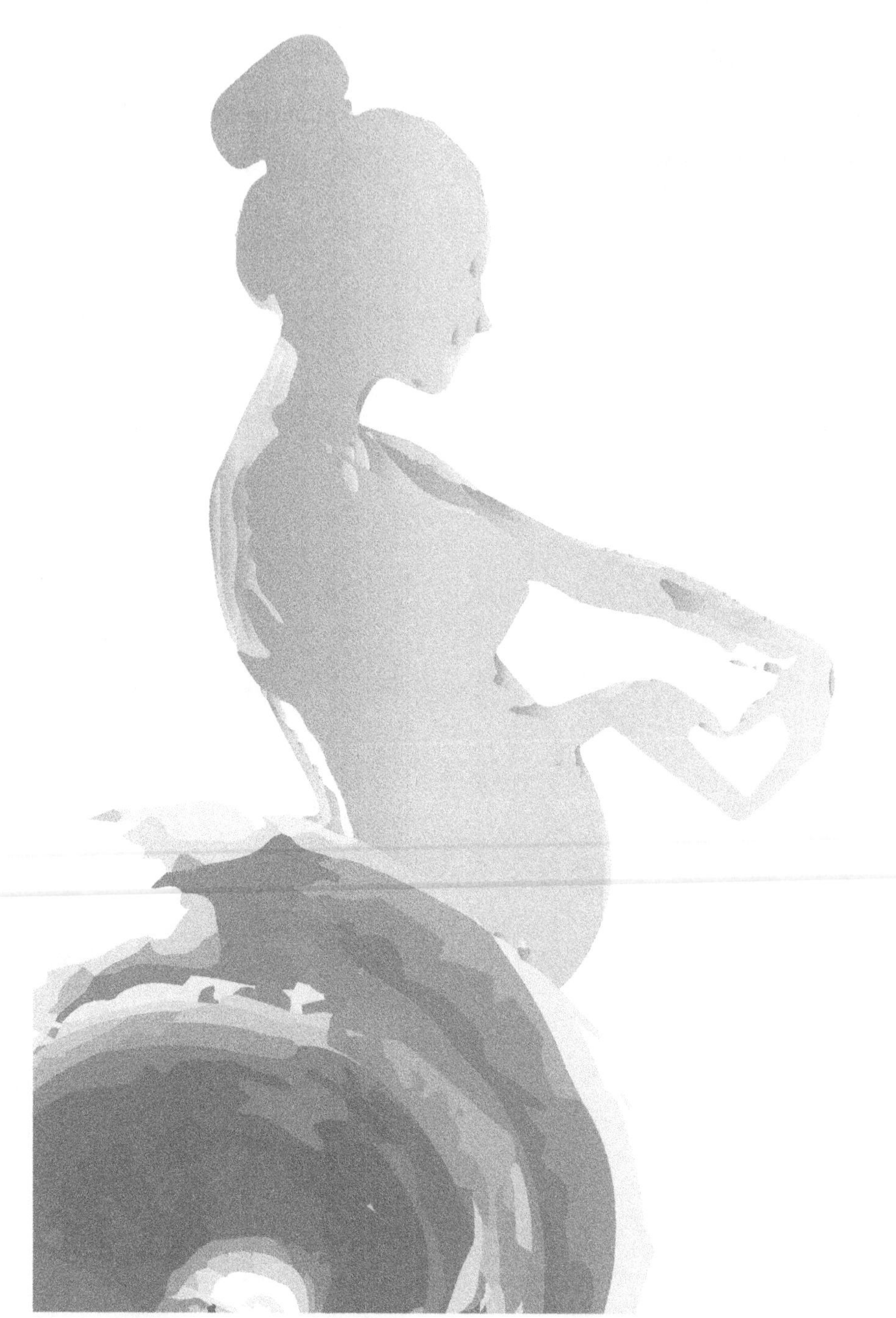

Chapter 3: It's time! It's time!

Letter to my unborn baby

Dear Arielito:

I suspect you will look a lot like me physically. You will inherit my plump complexion, brown eyes, straight black hair... From your daddy, you will get long limbs, cinematic eyelashes, a mischievous look, and a patience-killing hyperactivity that, just in case, you will also get from your two closest uncles.

From your maternal grandmother, if you don't inherit her energy and ability, I will inject it into you. I do not accept refusal in this inheritance of the Milan. And from your paternal grandmother, let's hope you absorb all the intelligence and dedication she puts into the family and into every professional project.

From your maternal grandfather, I hope you also inherited that, as well as his green eyes, but you know... I already googled those genetic things and you have a 75% chance of getting brown eyes. And from your paternal grandfather, you must have that unheard of talent for craftsmanship. Again, I'm not going to take no for an answer.

There are other people who do not belong to our family, but whom I have known in my 30 years of life and whom I call "friends", from whom I would like you to take qualities. But since genetics has no influence there, I will let you learn by meeting them and traveling ... because they are scattered. You will have no choice.

In December, I'll check you out to see if my imagination was right.... Or if you are so much more than I could have imagined while waiting for you to be born.

Speaking of which, are you okay? Sometimes I imagine you're already uncomfortable in there. I say this because of the jerky, repetitive way you move, as if you are asking for the big space that awaits you in the crib.

Your movements are like messages, the most visible way you communicate with me in the morning after I drink the milk prepared by Grandpa Wilfre, who also prepares our lunches and meals, after which you always make my belly ripple as if you were saying a resounding thank you.

Too bad not everyone has the patience to watch you dance in there over and over again, because - I have to tell you - sometimes you take too long to repeat the steps. Only Grandma Meylin and Aunt Rosy take the risk of waiting next to your belly until you react, even though they spend 24 hours a day doing it. They are inexhaustible when it comes to you.

I imagine that you dance when you are happy. But there are other circumstances, almost always at night, when I suspect you are protesting. Why do you protest? Do you remember that you were not born?

In these 38 weeks together, I have gotten to know you a little.

For example, I know that since I was about 20 weeks old, you didn't like me working. You found my work chair unbearable and kicked me in the ribs to tell me to please shorten my workday. You disliked the 11:00 a.m. editorial tips; I guess because they always delayed your feeding. I would always give your message to my boss, you could ask her later.....

I also discovered that the noise annoyed you. The Brazilian soap opera, due to the high volume of the television that the grandparents insist on keeping on, upsets you. Just like the sounds of Grandma Elsa when she gives us one of her usual "mommy fights", although in this case I think you are defending me. Don't worry, you'll have time to receive them, too, and just so you know, they're out of love. Protection is not necessary.

Another finding is the certainty that you love chocolate...but you have caused me to dislike it. You become too intense when I give it to you, and you don't let me sleep! Speaking of sleep... you don't get much rest to speak of. Before, when you had less time in there, you were unnoticeable, but now, unless you're a bit of a sleepwalker, you only lie quietly between 2:00 and 9:00 in the morning.

Do you plan to keep up this pace when you are born? Poor daddy, who works all day long and has to help mommy get out of bed or get into bed hundreds of times to convince you to stay still. From your nocturnal behavior, I deduce that you don't like our bed very much, which at least reassures me... because your crib cannot be left without an inhabitant. It is dangerous for you to sleep with mommy and daddy.

My long-awaited baby, I'm going to finish. I dare you to defy my imagination and come out any way you want... even Chinese, if that was the family gene you grabbed when you formed. Surprise us with your arrival, but don't hesitate. I am desperate. I have hours and days to spare. I can't bear to wait another second of my life to devote myself to you out here.

40 weeks: This Body Is Not Yours

I feel that my body is not mine. When I look at myself in the mirror these days, I see myself as a kind of desperate human container. And contrary to what I suspected, my baby does not seem to be in a hurry to get out.

He's moving intensely, with force, as if at any moment he's going to break that kind of bag that separates him from the ultimate exit to the outside world, but he doesn't. ....

Either he doesn't have the strength, or he doesn't feel like it, or he's too comfortable.

There is something strange about reaching 40 weeks of pregnancy. You imagine that the baby should already be with the family, especially since in most anecdotes heard in the doctor's office or polyclinic almost all pregnant women gave birth in the 38th or 39th week of pregnancy.

It is only when you go to the Pregnancy Consultation at Term, at the Maternity Hospital that you realize that it is normal to be in your 40 weeks without anything happening. There, in line, all the girls are just like me: bursting at the seams with so much belly, and crazy to meet their little ones.

But we must be patient, says the doctor.

The last of these consultations was desperate, almost as desperate as the first one, the one in which they "beat" the C-section recommended by the orthopedist at 38 weeks of pregnancy.

This time I went, accompanied by my husband, with the secret hope that I would be admitted immediately to induce labor and meet my little one. But no. There are protocols that you do not know. For example, it has been established that if you have no risk factors - which is my case because, despite being overweight, I am "normotensive" and my blood sugar levels are in order - you can wait another week at home for the natural birth to take place.

In other words, I should not return until I reach 41 weeks... unless I am surprised by the symptoms that announce the arrival of a new citizen into the world.

The only good thing about this last visit to the maternity hospital was to see my baby again, thanks to the ultrasound. It was revealed to us that he was narrow due to the small space, and big, weighing 7.92 pounds. According to his father, if I ate a loaf of bread, he would immediately reach 8. He is also in the cephalic position, ready to brighten our lives with his arrival.

Now I do not dare to think about a possible birth date. I have been disappointed so many times that now I just wait... and imagine what family life will be like when he is here.

How will I organize my activities? What are the most immediate problems to solve after the birth? How will I make sure the wounds of childbirth heal quickly? Where will I find time for exercise and professional development? ....

Advice is welcome.

41 Questions I Asked Google and Doctors

Since I had just started my 41st week of pregnancy and the baby had not yet been born, I decided to give those who are or will be facing motherhood some of the most frequently asked questions that we all ask ourselves during these 9 months of waiting.

I found several answer in an excellent application, available on the internet, named Baby Center https://www.babycenter.com.

Here are the questions:

How long does a pregnancy last?

Why is the date of my last period so important?

Is there a way to know the exact day our baby was conceived?

What are the most common pregnancy symptoms?

Is it true that boys' bellies are different from girls' bellies?

Why do doctors take so long with pregnant women?

Do I have to have a vaginal exam every time I go to the doctor?

Is it logical to put speculums on pregnant women and won't it cause miscarriage?

Do pregnant women always have priority in consultations?

What are the main risk factors during pregnancy?

How much weight can I gain during pregnancy and what does it depend on?

What happens if I do not go to a consultation with the specialists?

Why should I carry a copy of my medical history with me?

Why do I need to be tested in each trimester of my pregnancy?

How does my blood group and my husband's blood group affect my pregnancy?

What family characteristics can my baby inherit?

What are the most common genetic diseases that can be inherited?

Why is a genetic ultrasound necessary?

Is it possible for my baby to be born with a malformation that is not detected by ultrasound?

How will I know my baby's sex?

Can doctors make a mistake in determining sex from an ultrasound?

Is vaginal discharge dangerous during these months?

How can I protect myself from vaginal infections?

Is it safe to have sex when I'm pregnant?

How late should I work?

Do I have any rights as a pregnant woman?

What are the most common aches and pains during pregnancy?

What can I take to help with backache and headaches?

What medications should a pregnant woman not take?

How often should I see an obstetrician during my pregnancy?

Why should I see a cardiologist after 24 weeks of pregnancy?

What should I do if I have pain in my lower abdomen?

What happens if there are blood spots?

When will I feel the baby move?

How will I know if my baby is moving enough?

Is it true that babies move less at the end of pregnancy?

What are the causes that put the baby's life at risk during pregnancy?

What types of births are there?

How will I know if I need a C-section?

What are the risks to the baby from natural childbirth and cesarean section?

What happens if my baby is born after 40 weeks?

Medical consultations near childbirth

Finally, my baby was born. On the 18th day of this December, 2018 - against all odds that had marked delivery for earlier dates - a team of obstetricians and gynecologists finally managed to get him out of my womb.

I was already 41.5 weeks pregnant, which meant we were dangerously close to the commonly accepted end of pregnancy limit. I was only two days away from the dreaded 42-week mark.

Fortunately, being admitted to the hospital made it easier for the doctors to keep a close eye on my progress, because when I went to the maternity hospital at 41 weeks for a Term Pregnancy Consultation, the doctor decided it was time for me to stay there.

Honestly, I will tell you that I already doubted the effectiveness of that consultation. This was the third time I had seen the specialist, and the "you're fine, come back next week" almost made me more desperate than the extension of my waiting period. Do the math: My due date was December 5, and Ariel was born on the 18th.

The first consultation was at 38 weeks, when an orthopedic specialist and the gynecologist at the family practice suggested to the hospital doctors the possibility of a C-section due to the scoliosis of more than 45 degrees of dorso-lumbar deviation that I have had since I was 11 years old.

At the consultation, I was sent to the optional vice-directorate of the maternity hospital, where I was told that the C-section would not be performed because the scoliosis pathology I suffered from did not qualify for surgery. Finally, I was told to return when I was 40 weeks pregnant.

I did so and was examined again. Again, I was advised to wait another week for contractions at home. On the day I was 41.1 weeks, after the third visit, I was admitted...but already in the hospital, the doctors kept repeating the same thing: let's wait for the pain.

To reassure myself, I told myself that a specialist would never put a baby's life at risk, and that if they made me wait until almost 42 weeks for the contractions to appear on their own, it was because their experience and knowledge had certified that it was not dangerous.

I can't say that this self-talk reassured me, because everything I read on Google told me otherwise. I could never shoo away the possibility of amniotic fluid leaking, my child having fetal distress, defecating in my belly, or changing the cephalic position he'd had since twenty and so weeks into a dangerous pelvic position. But I tried.

And luck was with me.

In the maternity hospital, I was placed in the K room, where there were 10 beds, almost all of them occupied by pregnant women suffering from complex pathologies, from which I felt free. For them, the fact that someone was there "just waiting to give birth" was something strange, because they had been admitted for several months to keep their illnesses under control.

In room K, I had follow-up ultrasounds every day until something went wrong.

The K-room and its little demons

Of all of my pregnant roommates, I remember only Roxana's name. Roxana is 16 years old and is waiting in Room K of the Maternity Hospital for the doctors to decide whether she will have a natural birth or a C-section when the time comes. She is 36 weeks pregnant, has epilepsy, and developed pre-eclampsia during her pregnancy.

Roxana is in bed 10. I am in bed 9. Since my admission, I have noticed that she is not only the youngest of all of us there, but also the one who is most afraid of the labor process and the one who interacts the least with the other patients. She is also the only one who has companions both day and night. She became pregnant when she was in the 9th grade, so, in the eyes of her family and doctors, she is a child despite her pregnancy.

I am writing this when I have been here for over 24 hours. I was admitted on a Friday, through the Term Pregnant Consult, because I was over 41 weeks pregnant and had no indication that my baby was going to be born... No contractions, no water breaking, no expulsion of mucus plug.

This hospital room is the closest thing to a school that I have experienced in 7 years. Of the 10 girls admitted, only two of us are ready to give birth at any time. We both know that we will be leaving soon. But there are others, the leaders of the girls, who still have a long time to spend between doctors, nurses, tests and quick visits from family members.

They are the last to go to bed, the ones who turn off the lights, the ones who generate the most interesting conversations, and the ones who bully the other pregnant women: those who were admitted for some small and ephemeral reason, or those who are disliked because of their appearance, their smell, their projection, or because they create an implicit competition for their sociability.

The reasons for their admission are the classic risk factors of pregnancy: there are diabetics, hypertensive patients, some who have been leaking amniotic fluid for weeks, the underage adolescent and one over 40 years of age.

It's interesting how life goes for people who spend almost 9 months of their pregnancy in a hospital. Unlike me, for whom it's more like a walk or something slightly better than being at home, where I was bored out of my mind, they wish they were at home with their other children, their husbands and their families.

I spent three days with them, enough time to learn and adapt to their routines, which are those of almost all patients who have not yet given birth.

Even if you don't want to, the nurses - whom you learn to love because of the number of hours they spend with us each shift - wake you up to take your blood pressure, hand out the prenatal pills and daily vitamins necessary for the baby to grow strong and well nourished.

You open your eyes, smile resignedly at them and follow their instructions, then slowly get up to go to the bathroom. There is always someone who stays in bed until 7:30 a.m., when it is no longer possible to sleep because life in the hospital is becoming more intense.

Around 8:30 a.m., the doctors hand in their shifts and check each patient in the room. Along with them are the students, who are asked from time to time about the ailments of pregnant women and how best to treat them. A sixth-year medical undergrad from Ghana was assigned to follow me from the time I was admitted.

He is friendly, but he doesn't inspire the same confidence in me as other classmates...or the doctors, for that matter. I try to overcome this insecurity by telling myself that I'm been influenced by a stigma, and that everyone deserves a chance to learn, even if I'm the one subjected to the experiment.

After the visits, there's not much to do except wait for noon, when the families "land" with small food fountains that, when uncovered, fill the room with the aromas of home.

And then to sleep again, all of them, as if hoping that when they close their eyes, time will speed up and the days or weeks left to meet their babies will pass quickly.

In the evening, family and nostalgia return, wrapped in the taste of steak, rice, beans and cookies. This is also the time when pregnant women take advantage of their visitors to carry the buckets of water to the bathroom that they cannot lift due to the size of their bellies, and to help them administer medications that they cannot take on their own.

Since there is no television, after the visits, one of the girls usually breaks the ice with a topic of conversation. The room leaders move from their beds to the bed of the one who started the conversation or invite her to their corner, while the others join in with anecdotes from their beds.

Night falls. There is nothing else to do. I throw myself on my bed, hoping to fall asleep, as do most of the girls, while the leaders go down the hall to visit former residents who have already given birth.

Around 6:30 a.m. the next day, in the hope that one of our babies will be born, the nurses return to give us the "wake up" call with their vitamins, prenatal pills, and end-of-watch vibe. It's an endless cycle that I broke at 41.4 weeks when I was told that the amniotic fluid in my belly had dropped from 8 to 4 and that could be dangerous at that point.

And then I was moved to another room.

Labor induction experience

On Monday, December 17, the day of Saint Lazarus, the Yoruba Orisha, the ultrasound corresponding to 41.4 weeks of pregnancy revealed a significant loss of amniotic fluid in my abdomen. I was not surprised. I assumed that something was going to happen because the pain associated with labor was taking too long to show up and I knew that the risks associated with a post-term delivery were increasing.

Immediately, the doctors in the K room of the maternity hospital decided that given the length of my pregnancy and what this loss could mean for my baby, it was time to transfer me to the Perinatal Care Unit, a more specialized place where they would keep a close eye on my baby's condition.

I only stayed in Perinatal Care until the next day, December 18, at 6:00 a.m., when the doctor on duty performed another ultrasound, which confirmed an even greater loss of amniotic fluid.

I had already been informed that if this were to happen, labor would be induced to speed up the birth that was naturally taking so long. I remained optimistic. Since I had been informed in my 38th week of pregnancy that my scoliosis did not qualify me for a C-section, I had psychologically prepared myself for this option, which should have been the first.

For someone who thought all her life that the day she decided to become a mother she would have a C-section, it was not easy to adjust to the idea of natural childbirth. In general, many girls are afraid of this moment. The intensity of the contractions is terrifying. That is why I began to search the Internet for information on how to make this process easier and what the advantages of this type of birth are.

Little by little, a C-section seemed to be the worst and most risky way to give birth.

On the day of the induction, December 18, I took a huge bath from head to toe, as our mothers advice. I was taken to the delivery room in a wheelchair, which was used in the hospital according to medical protocol. Once there, I said goodbye to my husband and the rest of my family to begin an experience that I found both terrifying and beautiful.

Upon entering the delivery room, you are given a green gown and each pregnant woman is warned that underwear is not necessary. Underwear gets in the way, the doctors simplify.

You walk down a hallway where you learn that there is a kind of "messenger nurse" through which the pregnant women, who can be there for up to 24 hours, send messages to their families stationed outside the room.

And when you get to the place where you will be induced, you will see some beds where several pregnant women are lying, connected to a monitor that shows the heart rate of the babies and the contractions of the mothers. On a table there are at least four or five doctors who read thoroughly not only the medical history of the mother, but also the card of each pregnant woman.

Until that moment, I believe that, with the exception of me, no one had ever read in such detail what had been written by each doctor I had seen during my pregnancy.

After reading and asking for details, they called the head nurse, who told the other nurses to prepare different induction serums with oxytocin. Special ones for the three diabetics and the hypertensive who came with me, and a normal one for me. They channeled our veins and right after that a doctor told us to accompany her to check our vaginas. This doctor broke my water.

Minutes later, as if in déjà vu, I was lying on one of the pre-natal beds, hooked up to the monitor that allowed me to monitor my baby's heartbeat and my almost non-existent contractions.

While I was in that room, the heart of the maternity ward, I witnessed many stories, such as that of the 16-year-old girl whose pregnancy was uptake at 30 weeks, sending the team of doctors on duty that day scrambling because much of the girl's follow-up data was missing.

I even came close to seeing a baby born in front of my eyes when one of the girls came in so much pain that while the doctors were attaching the monitor to her, she was pushing for her baby to be born. Thirty minutes later I saw her happily holding her baby.

One of the great advantages of some maternity hospitals in Cuba is that they allow the fathers to participate in the delivery process. So, five hours after the induction, my husband, dressed in green from head to toe, came to see me.

That was one of the best moments of the day. The second was when they placed my tiny baby next to me on the bed in the recovery room where I was staying after an emergency C-section, indicated because of the fetal distress showed on the monitor and the precarious condition of my body for natural childbirth.

The doctor who performed my C-section later told me that when she went to remove the child, she touched my deformed spine. "You would never have delivered naturally," she assured me.

7 tips on how to prepare for labor

They say at home that I am addicted to the Internet, and I correct them: I am addicted to searching for information...in any medium. What happens is that it is so, so easy to find information on the Internet that the temptation to dig there instead of going to a book or a specialist is overwhelming.

Since I don't see this as a problem, my first piece of advice to any girl facing pregnancy for the first time would be:

Learn as much as you can about your options.

Many people often recommend that you don't seek out information about different birth options so as not to be traumatized. This advice hasn't worked for me. I prefer to know what I am going to face, and so from the time I arrived at 36 weeks of pregnancy, I started getting information about how to know if I was going to go into labor, how many days I would have to give birth after my water broke or my mucus plug came out, or what the possible risks were of my baby reaching 42 weeks in the womb...which almost happened.

Explore the benefits of natural childbirth

I have to admit that before 36 weeks, I tried not to think too much about what was going to happen at the end of my pregnancy. I focused on enjoying my growing belly, but when the time came that my baby would soon surprise me with his arrival into the world, I began to become aware of the benefits of natural childbirth.

Like most girls, I wanted a C-section, but the doctors said that was not one of my options, so I started looking for data on the benefits of natural childbirth, and guess what? There are many.

For starters, you get your baby right after birth, they say your milk comes in faster, and the recovery process is just a few days and not more than 40 days like with a C-section, you are spared the huge wound in your abdomen with its possibilities of infection or ending up with a hernia, and you can be discharged from the hospital much faster.

Learn exercises to make the birth process easier.

When I was in the delivery room, one of the doctors said that pregnant women should take some classes to make this process easier. She called it "Puericulture". My doctor never informed me that this existed, so I arrived at the maternity hospital knowing nothing about how to give birth except for the basics: opening my legs and pushing when I felt contractions.

Good advice: learn how to control your breathing, how to count contractions, how to control pain, and which side to lie on, among other tactics that will make the moment of your baby's birth more bearable.

Don't get married to the idea that a C-section is better.

Thinking that a C-section is the best option is a mistake, and I am not saying this because I have benefited from it. I came close to giving birth naturally, and I would have if my child's life had not been in danger. The female body is designed to give birth to life. Mentalize that and it will be easier for you.

Learn the facts about recovery and the risks of surgery.

Preparing for a C-section is the same as preparing for any other surgery, with the notable difference that two lives are at risk. You will experience the stress of being in the operating room, the anesthesia as it numbs you or may not work as it should, the opening and closing of the incision, the pain of the wound, the almost inability to move when they put your baby next to you, a longer and more painful recovery than with natural childbirth, having to wait more than 40 days to resume your normal life and almost three months to return to exercise...in short. Prepare yourself psychologically to follow the recommendations and ask your family for support because you will need it.

Try not to listen to other birth stories

Well, some friends told me not to pay too much attention to the anecdotes about childbirth that I would hear in the doctor's office. Some girls give birth very quickly, while others have very traumatic stories. Some are desperate to have a C-section and others are just as desperate to have a natural birth.

If there's one thing I can recommend, it's the same thing I was told: don't be traumatized by other people's stories. Always think positive, although in the maternity hospital you should always keep an eye on what the doctors say about the evolution of your condition.

Suggest enjoying the road to birth as an adventure.

That's how I approached it. I thought that even if I wanted to have another baby, it might be not only my first but also my only child, so I would try to enjoy every step of the way to childbirth in a way that would leave me with a good memory forever. That would be my best advice.

If you have to push, push hard. If you have to breathe, breathe hard. If you have to endure pain, try all the time with as much energy and optimism as you can. When you see his little face, you will understand that it was all worth it.

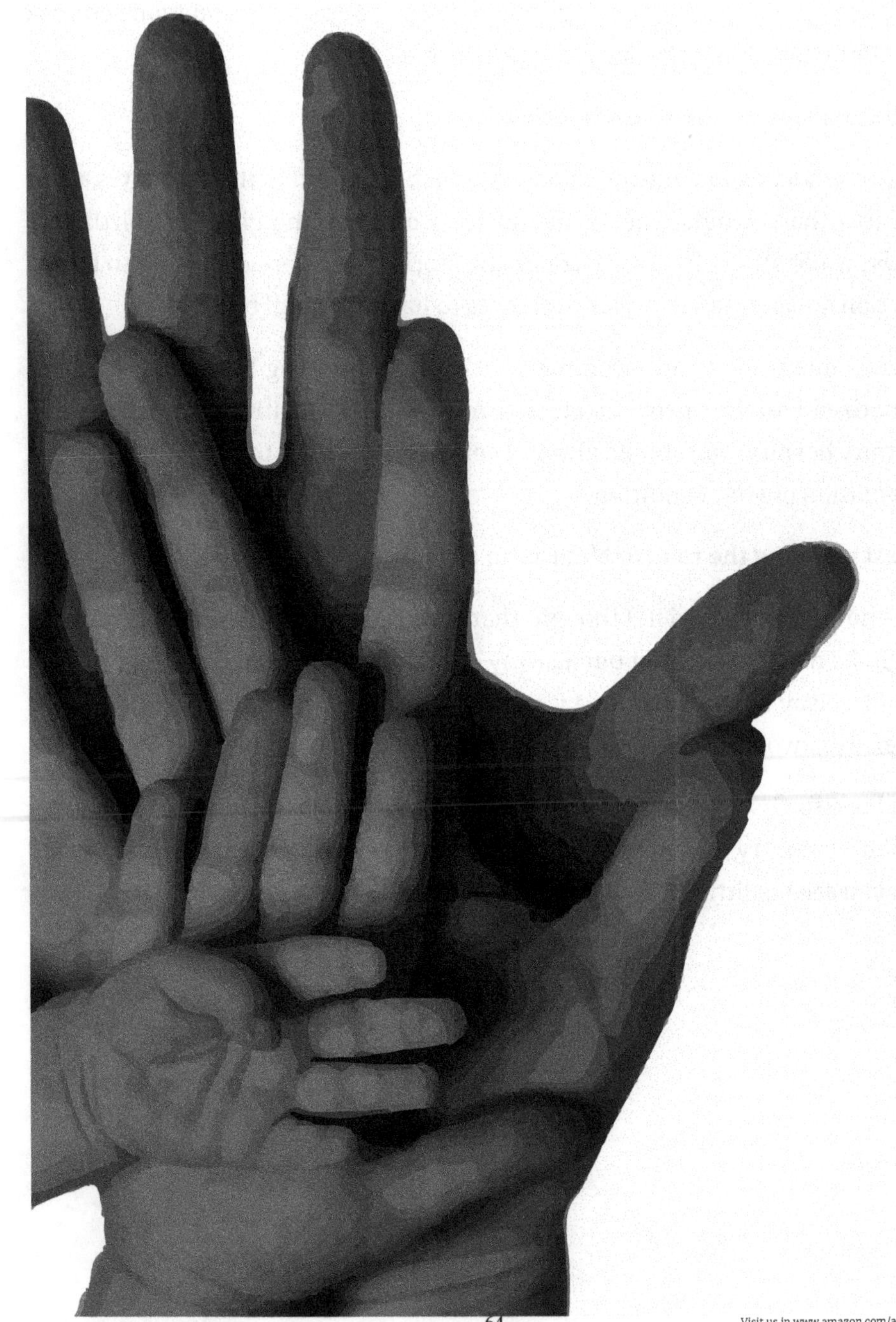

Chapter 4: Arielito

Birth

I have a video of my baby being born. It shows the hands of the obstetrician who delivered him as she opens the wound in my abdomen just enough to fit the tiny head of my baby, born asleep, through the opening.

With impressive technique, she cleans his nostrils and mouth while the rest of his body is still inside me, and finally pulls him out completely. He was born asleep. Some in the family say he must have spent more or less the entire pregnancy that way, since he was born at 41.5 weeks and didn't make the slightest effort to come out on his own.

I also have a video of his first cry, right there in the operating room, although the doctor says the first thing Ariel did was sneeze.

I cannot deny that I am proud of the result of the fusion of my genes and those of my love.

The child is not what I imagined, but he is superior. And every time I look at him, I am convinced that it was worth every second of pain from the contractions caused by the induction of labor, and even the panic attack that the C-section caused me, the discomfort of the IV and the catheter, and the painful and long recovery after the surgery.

When the doctor informed me that my baby couldn't be born naturally, I was not afraid. All my life I thought it would be a cesarean section because of the severe scoliosis that kept my spine in a cast for six years. Then I had to prepare myself psychologically for the possibility of vaginal birth, and that was an extra effort.

So now I faced the need for surgery as something that was destined for me, although in the end, it was because of an Uneasy Fetal Status (IFS) and not because of my historical scoliosis.

Through glass panes in the ceiling of the operating room, due to the curious placement of the lamps about them, the entire operation could be observed. But I did not look up. I preferred to be blind, just listening to the conversation of the doctors who talked about the human and the divine, without taking an eye off me.

Then came the transfer from one stretcher to another to take me from the operating room to the recovery room. I had to help them move me a little, using my shoulders as a lever, because my 29 extra pounds, in addition to the 176 I already weighed before pregnancy, were too much for the doctors.

Having a cesarean section is not "pretty" or easy. It is a serious invasion of a woman's body that leaves her limp, bleeding and in pain for days.

Fortunately, a few minutes after the operation, in the recovery room, the bed that will witness the first encounter with their babies awaits all mothers.

According to medical protocol, as soon as I entered, a nurse placed my baby in the crib. I couldn't see him because the crib was too high, so I was dying of curiosity. Ten minutes later, she returned and carefully placed him next to me.

In the information room, the whole family waited expectantly for news about the birth and me. Until the doctors brought the baby to them before placing him next to me.

The first month

I write so as not to forget. At this stage of motherhood, I have little time for anything but taking care of the little one. He can't live without me and I don't want to live without him.

The first month was the most stressful of my life. Today my husband jokes that I didn't want to leave the hospital, but what can you do when you don't know what is good or bad for your baby, when Google says one thing and the doctors say another?

The first crisis was in the recovery room after the C-section when I felt my little son sneeze once, twice, three, even six or seven times. I was so worried, lying there on the bed with the veins running and the wound in my belly, hardly able to caress the little one, that I called the nurse to find out if the sneezing was normal. She said it was.

I would later learn that Arielito was sneezing for the first time in his life, before he even cried.

Four days after the C-section, we were discharged and went home. Then came the second crisis: the umbilical cord.

It was supposed to fall off by itself after 10 days and we were supposed to clean it with alcohol every day... but Arielito's umbilical cord was still attached to his skin after 10 days of birth and it smelled bad. As you can imagine, at my instigation, we ended up at the doctor's office, where Valentina (remember my nurse?) cleaned the little navel like she was from another world.

Seeing that I was not satisfied, the gynecologist who was consulting that day referred us to the neonatology department of the children's hospital in our area, just in case, the gynecologist referred us to the neonatology department of the pediatric hospital in our area. And there we took Arielito in his baby trolley for his first big walk around town. At the hospital, they cleaned the umbilicus again and told us about the silver nitrate treatment that they offer in cases of infection, but recommended that we wait a few more days. The next morning the umbilicus came out.

I did not realize how anxious I could be until I was faced with his first congestion at 15 or 16 days after been born. The stress took over me, the room, the house... I was haunted by the possibility that my baby might choke. That I wouldn't be there to help him in a moment of suffocation.

Grandparents

There are grandparents and grandparents.

As far as I can remember, I lived alone with my father, mother, and sister for most of my life. My grandparents lived in houses far away from mine, although in the same province, so my relationship with them was loving but distant. My cousins who grew up nearby were more fortunate.

We knew only one of our great-grandparents, who died when we were young… And of my grandparents' siblings, we occasionally heard anecdotes or were introduced to one of them because they happened to be in the same place as my parents.

I don't remember my grandparents giving us many presents. On the contrary, it was my sister and I who religiously gave them presents every birthday. We also visited them on weekends and holidays. Now only one of them is alive, my maternal grandmother, with whom the relationship grew closer over the years, and both my sister and I became aware of the value of family when it is so large and vital.

My baby's story will not be like ours.

Since the news of the pregnancy spread, my mother doesn't know what to do with so much joy. She wants to double everything: the crib, the diapers, the sheets, the clothes, the bottles… she would double the baby and me if she could, to have us with her 24 hours a day. This will be her first grandchild, but she is already thinking about the second ("because there has to be a second," she says) and my younger sister's future offspring. She has become a specialist in obtaining essential parenting supplies at unbelievably low prices.

The paternal grandmother, who has already had her first experience with my little nephew Thiago, has a briefcase full of advice and creative ideas. Her specialty is solving problems: Snacks? "The ones from my job"; Money? "I'll help you"; Lots of antiseptic fabric but not enough crib diapers? "I know someone who can sew them"; Is your job far from the kindergarten? "I met a caregiver"; What's missing from the layette? "They sell it in such and such a place…" Her activism is often contagious…although it's hard to shake my patience to search and shop only when I feel it's time.

The paternal grandfather is enthusiastic about everything related to the future newborn. He lovingly prepares breakfasts and meals according to the rhythm of my growing belly, and when I wash the miniature clothes, he enjoys counting each tiny outfit to show how rich the little one's wardrobe will be. With patience, she has repaired every wooden object that will support the baby's life: cribs (double, as I already explained), closet, feeding chairs, little horse, etc....

Try as I might, I can't imagine how my father, who died when I was 16, would relate to my baby. It is very difficult to project an image of a grandfather when that of a father was cut off... but to compensate, I have the peace of mind that Arielito will be born with extra grandparents.

For example, he has my mother-in-law's sister and her husband: Justo and Marlen, who for no reason would accept to be called aunts and uncles, nor great uncles, they are not. Their microfamily is so close to my husband's microfamily that Ariel cannot be less than a grandchild. And so this grandmother in particular has been on top of the layette, the search for what's missing, my health and the babie's... The last thing she did was to send me a list of all the phone numbers where she could be reached the moment my water broke.

I can't wait to see all five of them when I give birth. They each have their own theory of what the child will be like and how it should be raised. .... I'll let you know.

On our first night together

What would babies say, if they could, about that first encounter with their mothers? Ariel Alejandro, if asked, might say that from what little he could see between nap and nap, his mother looked tired. She was disheveled, her eyes half-closed, and she wore a green cap stained with blood. She didn't look very pretty, but she had such a wide, permanent smile that it was impossible to pay attention to anything else...not even her breasts.

That first night he and I spent together was one of the most beautiful and intense of my 30 years. And it wasn't my best day. Between the blood stains from the surgery and the "bleeding" coming out like some sort of menstruation, the annoying urinary catheter, and the endless saline solution attached to one of the veins in my left hand, the six hours I would be in the recovery room seemed endless.

Until they put my baby next to me...

After nine months of waiting, we finally met. Of course, I didn't expect it to be in this condition. The pain in the wound hardly allowed me to move to look at his face or offer him my breast. I was a little scared. How could I take care of him for six hours when I was almost immobile? To make matters worse, the nurse in the room kept reminding me not to lift my head...or I would jeopardize the outcome of the surgery.

So I settled into that personal bed as best I could and took in as much of my wide-eyed baby as I could. He was a slant-eyed little boy, with straight hair and plenty of it on his head, back, and arms. A handmade handle on his left arm told me what no one had told me until that moment: he had been born at 4:30 p.m. on that December 18, 2018, and weighed 7.13 pounds.

7.13 pounds! The whole family thought he would be much more, and that was reflected in the clothes he was wearing, too big for him: a little white shirt with long sleeves and a pair of light blue one-piece little pants. Seeing him like that made me smile mischievously, because when I thought about it, everything fit him like pajamas.

With his pupils dilated and of an indecipherable color, Ariel stared intently at my face. And he sneezed a lot. I called the nurse and she said it was normal. Then, she asked me if I was a first-timer and my age. "30 years old," I told her. She added, "You waited too long." "I waited just the right time" I replied with a smile.

The nurse left and I turned my attention back to Ariel, who was now stretching his little neck and holding his head up with his mouth open. Following my instinct, I put a breast to his lips and he squeezed and sucked for the first time.

Would he get anything out? I had the impression that he would not, but he sucked relentlessly until he fell asleep. Then he would wake up just to pick up where he left off.

Around 11:00 p.m. I was informed that I would be spending the night in Recovery because there were no beds available in the hospital postpartum ward. I asked the nurse to call Information so they could orient my family, who were expecting my transfer at 1:00 a.m. She didn't. Should she have? I think she should have.

In all the maternity wards I went through, the medical staff was attentive to my family, but now I had to wait until my husband came upstairs worried at 1:00 a.m. and asked a nurse to ask for me. Only then did he know that I would not be moved until the morning.

I couldn't believe I had made it through the night. Sleepless and insomniac, afraid I would crush my baby, or that he would need me and I couldn't listen to him. The lights and sounds of the room, with all the medical staff available for emergency C-sections running through it, did not help me rest either.

In short, I spent almost 17 hours (out of 6) in the isolated recovery room. Alone with my newborn. It was not until 10:00 a.m. on December 19 that I was transferred to Room A, bed 19, where everyone was waiting for us in a festive mood to welcome the new life.

What I know about my little boy after 1 year together

On December 18, 2018, I became a mother, my most intense, exhausting and rewarding profession.

I am the mother of naughty Arielito, one year old, 2.44 feet tall, 26.01 pounds of weight, and inexhaustible energies that seem to take a worthy course at night.

I'll let you in on a secret: he's been sleeping from 8:00 p.m. to 4:30 a.m. for 4 days now… almost without interruption. Victory!

What I know about my little boy after 1 year together:

He loves to play and is very naughty.

He likes all kinds of food (and what is not food but edible too) but he prefers plantains, meat, beans, mommy's pudding, yogurt, bread, milk and…. cookies!

He gets very upset if he doesn't have his warm milk when he wakes up at 5 or 6 in the morning.

He is very independent. He prefers to do everything by himself: eating, brushing his hair, bathing, and learning to walk.

He loves to dance. He started dancing before he could walk.

He is very curious.

His logical thinking is very developed. He observes and reproduces. He disassembles and reassembles. He develops strategies to avoid obstacles.

His cousin Thiago, mom, dad, his aunt Hildita and his grandparents arouse in him an unbearable desire to nibble and cuddle.

He prefers his parents' bed to his crib or the baby trolley.

He knows his grandmother Elsa's house so well that he explodes with joy when he sees her house around the corner.

He was exclusively breastfed for 6 months (not even water), has teeth and has been sitting since he was 4 months old, crawled since he was 5, stood up on his own for the first time at 6, and walked alone at 11.

His first word was Yisi and he loves me.

Letter to Arielito on his first birthday

My little son,

We know you're growing up fast, and that one day you won't remember your first 365 days with Mommy and Daddy.

But we also know that one day you'll want to know.

You will want to know where you came from, and we will tell you about our romantic nights; about the growing belly; about how you traveled to Peru; about how you danced with a world champion wrestler when you were just an embryo; and about how you met an Internet challenge almost at the time of your birth (the video of pregnant women dancing!).

You'll want to know how your arrival in this world was, and who helped you be born when you still couldn't bring yourself to come out at 41.5 weeks.

You'll want to know what the people who love you most in life were like when you were a baby, and they were young and vibrant.

You'll want to know where your roots are in Cuba.

You will want to know when your first teeth came out, if you crawled or walked, what you were like, what you did, if you were a happy, mischievous, playful child...

You will want to know about your "mommy sickness" and "daddy sickness", and about the stumbles and learnings of your parents, who were learning every day with your master classes in never-never-ever sleep at any time, and pee, poop, pukes, diapers, boobs, and bottles.

You might even want to know why we're enthusiastic to celebrate your birthday even though everyone says you won't remember it,

And then, my little one, we can tell you because we love you and because every December is our birthday too.

Thanks to everyone who loves Arielito, and to his mommy and daddy, grandparents, aunts and uncles, and so on..., for joining us on this 1 year journey.

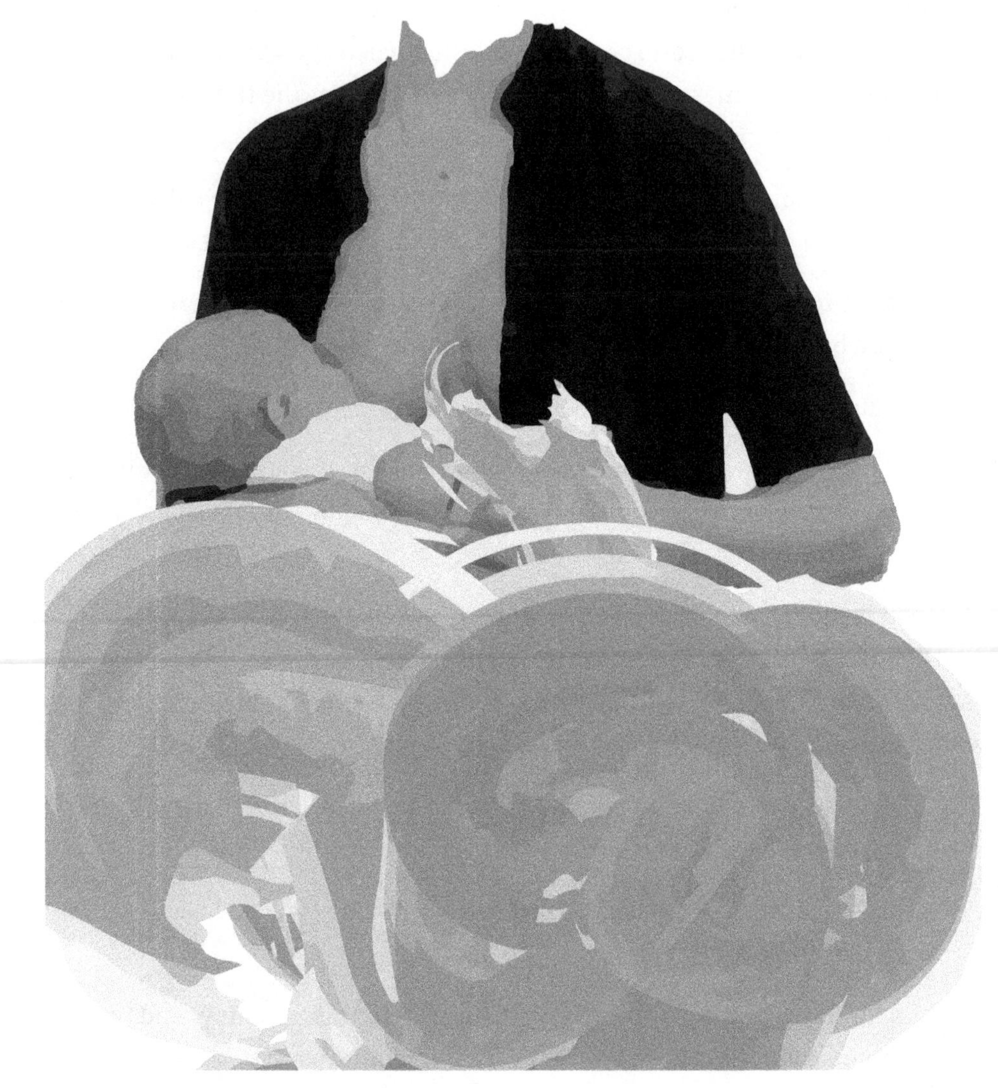

Journalist and web editor. Graduate in journalism at Oriente University, in Santiago de Cuba. Head of the Multimedia Department of the Granma Journal. Co-author of the ebook "Unfiltered Maternity".

Specialized in hypermedia journalism, social network management, web positioning, digital audience research and coordination of teams for these scenarios.

Member of the Hermanos Saiz Association and the Union of Journalists of Cuba. She has published in several digital and print magazines in Cuba and abroad.

Winner of digital journalism competitions in Cuba. She has made international press coverage in several countries, including Panama, Dominican Republic and Peru.